Wilms' Tumor

WILMS' TUMOR

Edited by

CARL POCHEDLY, M.D.
Nassau County Medical Center
East Meadow, New York

DENIS MILLER, M.D.
New York Hospital
Cornell Medical Center
New York, New York

With Introduction by

JERRY Z. FINKLESTEIN, M.D.
UCLA School of Medicine
Harbor General Hospital
Torrance, California

A WILEY BIOMEDICAL PUBLICATION

JOHN WILEY & SONS, New York ● London ● Sydney ● Toronto

Library of Congress Cataloging in Publication Data

Main entry under title:

Wilms' tumor.

    (A Wiley biomedical publication)
    Includes bibliographical references and index.
    1. Nephroblastoma. I. Pochedly, Carl. II. Miller,
Denis R. [DNLM: 1. Nephroblastom. WJ358 W744]
RC280.K5W54   618.9′29′9461   75-37983
ISBN 0-471-69137-2

Contributors

Pierre Burtin, M.D., Ph.D., Head of the Immunochemistry Laboratory and Associate Director, Institut de Recherches Scientifiques sur le Cancer, Villejuif, France

J. R. Cope, M.D., R.D., M.B., Consultant Radiologist, Southport and Ornskirt Hospitals, Lancashire, England

Harry S. David, M.D., Chief Resident (Urology), St. Luke's Hospital Center, Visiting Clinical Fellow (Urology), College of Physicians and Surgeons, Columbia University, and Department of Urology, St. Luke's Hospital Center, New York, New York

Jerry Z. Finklestein, M.D., Associate Professor of Pediatrics, UCLA School of Medicine, Chief, Division of Pediatric Hematology-Oncology, Harbor General Hospital, Torrance, California

Joseph Giangiacomo, M.D., Assistant Professor of Pediatrics, Pediatric Nephrology, St. Louis University School of Medicine, Cardinal Glennon Memorial Hospital for Children, St. Louis, Missouri

Phillip Holland, M.D., Professor of Pediatrics, School of Medicine, University of Kentucky, Lexington, Kentucky

D. W. O'Gorman Hughes, M.D., M.B., B.S., F.R.A.C.P., Chairman, Division of Pediatric Haematology and Oncology, The Prince of Wales Hospital, Senior Lecturer in Pediatrics, University of New South Wales, Sydney, N.S.W., Australia

John M. Kissane, M.D., Professor of Pathology, Washington University School of Medicine, Associate Pathologist, Barnes and Affiliated Hospitals and St. Louis Children's Hospital, St. Louis, Missouri

Alfred A. de Lorimier, M.D., Pediatric Surgical Service, Associate Professor, Department of Surgery, School of Medicine, University of California, San Francisco, California

E. C. Pirtle, M.D., Ph.D., Microbiologist, Virological Research Laboratory, National Animal Disease Center, North Central Region, Agricultural Research Service, United States Department of Agriculture, Ames, Iowa

Louise C. Strong, M.D., Assistant Professor of Medical Genetics, Department of Biology, Health Service Center, Graduate School of Biomedical Sciences, Houston, Texas, and Consultant in Medical Genetics, Departments of Pediatrics and Medicine, M.D. Anderson Hospital and Tumor Institute, System Cancer Center, Houston, Texas

Melvin Tefft, M.D., Attending Radiotherapist, Memorial Hospital for Cancer and Allied Diseases, Professor of Radiology, Cornell University Medical College, New York, New York

H. Joachim Wigger, M.D., Associate Professor of Clinical Pediatric Pathology, College of Physicians and Surgeons, Columbia University and Associate Attending Pathologist, Division of Developmental Pathology, Presbyterian Hospital, New York, New York

James A. Wolff, M.D., Professor of Pediatrics, College of Physicians and Surgeons, Columbia University, New York, New York, and Attending Physician, Babies Hospital, The Children's Medical and Surgical Center of New York, New York, New York

D. G. Young, M.D., M.B., B.S., Department of Pediatric Surgery, Royal Hospital for Sick Children, Senior Lecturer, University of Glasgow, Yorkhill, Glasgow, Scotland

Preface

The extraordinary improvement in the results of treatment of Wilms' tumor has made it a model for the treatment of other childhood malignancies. The steady advances in the long-term survival rate of children with this tumor have done much to dispel pessimism and have spawned a new era of cautious optimism. Wilms' tumor is a symbol of hope that improvement in the results of treatment of other childhood malignancies may also be forthcoming.

Wilms' tumor is of particular interest to the pediatrician, surgeon, and oncologist for two major reasons. First, of all the childhood malignancies this tumor has the greatest potential for cure, even when metastases are present. Second, its management exemplifies the combined roles of surgery, radiotherapy, and chemotherapy. Advances in treatment over the past decade have further improved the survival rate for patients with Wilms' tumor. This increased survival rate depends mainly on early detection of the tumor by the general practitioner or pediatrician and the subsequent coordinated efforts of the surgeon, pathologist, radiotherapist, and chemotherapist. Improved preoperative management, precise initial determination of the extent of the disease, and detailed clinical evaluation of the patient following definitive therapy are very important.

Wilms' tumor is also important in the broader biologic sense because it is known to occur both in man and in many of the lower animals. The embryonal origin of Wilms' tumor has opened up another fascinating area for investigation of the pathogenesis and genetics of this tumor.

The primary purpose of this book is to survey in depth the biologic and clinical behavior of Wilms' tumor. The many significant advances in recent years on the fundamental nature of Wilms' tumor justify the publication of such a comprehensive monograph, the first on Wilms' tumor to be published. The second purpose of this book is to provide an up-to-date compendium on the optimal management of this disease for practicing physicians.

This book was designed and edited as a close collaborative effort between Dr. Finklestein and ourselves. Dr. Finklestein helped to select the topics and authors and approved the scientific content of each chapter. Together we edited the manuscripts to decide upon needed revisions and additions. Drs. Robert A. Price and Anthony Shaw reviewed the chapters that were relevant to their specialties, histopathology (Chapter 6) and surgery (Chapter 10).

We are very pleased to have been able to assemble an outstanding international team of oncologists to participate in the preparation of this important monograph. We are grateful also to our editors at John Wiley & Sons, Ms. Ruth Wreschner, and Mr. Alan Frankenfield, who provided a constant source of help and encouragement.

East Meadow, New York   CARL POCHEDLY, M.D.
New York, New York   DENIS R. MILLER, M.D.
September 1975

Contents

Wilms' Tumor

CHAPTER ONE

Introduction: Historical Review of Wilms' Tumor

JERRY Z. FINKLESTEIN, M.D.

Associate Professor of Pediatrics
UCLA School of Medicine
Chief, Division of Pediatric Hematology-Oncology
Harbor General Hospital
Torrance, California

Supported in part by grant CA 146560 from the National Cancer Institute.

With early diagnosis and treatment, Wilms' tumors can now be cured in the vast majority of cases. The history of Wilms' tumor is a therapeutic success story worth telling because of the encouragement it provides regarding treatment of childhood tumors, against which present-day therapeutic modalities are less effective. Wilms' tumor is an excellent subject for a monograph in pediatric oncology because it illustrates how successful therapy can be attained by physicians who work together as a team in treating the child with a complex disease.

Although Max Wilms published his classic monograph in 1899,[1] renal tumors of children that were presumably Wilms' tumor had been recognized much earlier in the medical literature in articles written by Rance in 1814[2] and Gairdner in 1828.[3] The first clinical description of renal cancer in a child was that of Van der Byl in *Lancet* in 1856.[4] Although his patient had an enormous tumor, one must doubt whether it was Wilms' tumor because of the long 7-year history. Nevertheless, his description of the patient is of interest as it relates the course of an untreated renal tumor in a young boy.

> The child's abdomen, soon after birth, became larger on the left side than on the right. It continued to increase in size very gradually until six months before his admission into the hospital, but it grew very rapidly afterwards. When he was admitted, the abdomen was much enlarged and crossed by large, tortuous veins. Enlargement existed especially on the left side and was produced by a tumour about eight inches in diameter. The tumour was slightly moveable, semi-elastic in some parts, and not painful on being handled. The intestines were felt over the edge of it on the right side. Four months after admission he walked a short distance, but had to be carried back to bed. He occasionally complained of great pain in the abdomen, which increased so much in size that he was soon unable to leave his bed; but he lingered on for months. His appetite was generally good, and his bowels regular; but he became gradually very thin, and died from exhaustion about 10 months after admission.

A postmortem examination performed by Van der Byl revealed a tumor originating from the left kidney. Unfortunately, the microscopic study was not complete.

By the mid-1800s it became apparent that children were dying of tumors of the kidney and that therapy was needed. On June 16, 1877, the first nephrectomy in a child was performed by Mr. Jessop at the Leeds Infirmary. The operation was described in *Lancet* 9 days later.[5] Jessop treated a child who at the age of 2 years had symptoms consisting of hematuria and irritation of the bladder. The child

> lost flesh and became more and more pallid. About two months ago a rapidly increasing tumor was discovered in the left renal region, and as the indications were those of malignant growth, Mr. Jessop determined to cut down upon it, and, if possible, to remove it. The incision was similar to that recommended for colotomy, but longer. When the diseased mass was reached, the kidney was peeled by means of the fingers, and a whipcord ligature was passed around the vessels and ureter, and firmly tied. The remainder of the growth was afterwards stripped away, and the

3

whipcord left to drain the wound. The operation was a formidable one owing to the large size of the diseased organ and the free venous haemorrhage which followed the separation of the growth from the surrounding structures. When removed the kidney weighed 16 ounces, and resembled encephaloid in appearance. The child was doing well on the 11th day. There was no peritonitis, the bowels acted freely, and the urine flowed abundantly, and was not stained. There was no vomiting, the temperature was but little above normal, and the child partook freely of milk.

Jessop's patient died 9 months later of metastases (reported by Czerny in 1888).[6]

The classic pathological description of what would later be called Wilms' tumor was written by Eberth in 1872,[7] who described a tumor in a 17-month-old girl who died 3 months after presentation. His description of the tumor's growth and pathology is in accord with the diagnosis of Wilms's tumor, and also represents the first well-documented histologic description. Three years later Cohnheim[8] described a congenital sarcoma of the kidney that fits into the classification of Wilms' tumor. Thus, by the late 1800s the disease had been categorized by the pathologists, and the institution of therapy had begun with the documentation of one successful nephrectomy.

In 1879 William Osler of McGill University in Montreal[9] provided the first noteworthy description by a North American. His paper recognized that the descriptions by Eberth,[7] Cohnheim,[8] Kocher and Langhans,[10] and others constituted a single, identifiable entity. Osler collected 4 cases from the literature and added 2 of his own. One patient was a 19-month-old boy who was found to have an incidental tumor on postmortem examination; the child had died from severe gastrointestinal symptomatology following a vaccination. A second patient was a 3-year-old girl who had a 6-week history of gastric and intestinal symptoms, occasional vomiting, and obstinate constipation. She had slight pain in the abdomen and, on inspection, a tumor was discovered in the left hypochondriac region just below the cartilage of the eighth rib. It was soft and apparently fluctuated. The child died suddenly, after getting up one morning and walking toward her mother's bed. Osler's pathologic description was most complete and agreed with what was eventually called Wilms' tumor. It is noteworthy that Osler collected the cases and grouped them together 20 years prior to Wilms' monograph. In 1894, Döderlein and Birch-Hirschfeld recognized that a variety of terms, namely, embryonal sarcoma, sarcoma of the kidney, adenomyosarcoma, and sarcoma musculare, were all used to designate the same tumor.[11] Wilms' tumor has also been called Birch-Hirschfeld's tumor in the older German literature.[6]

In the 1800s nephrectomies were considered major operations, with significant morbidity and mortality. The first large series of nephrectomies was reported by Israel in 1894.[12] He performed 37 operations for the following entities: malignant tumor 12; syphilis 2; tuberculosis 4; and hydronephrosis, pyelonephrosis, and kidney abscesses 19. Israel's operative mortality was 6 patients (16.2%). Two of his patients were 1 to 2 years of age; one died 5 months following surgery of liver metastases secondary to a "sarcoma of the kidney," while the other was well 11 months after operation.

By the end of the nineteenth century, embryonal sarcoma of the kidney had been recognized by Osler, and attempts at therapy had been initiated by Jessop and followed up by Israel. In 1899, Wilms' thoroughly reviewed the literature, and added 7 cases of his own to produce the definitive volume on the subject. [1]

The next major advance in therapy of Wilms' tumor occurred in 1915, when Alfred Friedlander of Cincinnati was presented with a patient who had an abdominal growth "so large that no surgeon was willing to undertake its removal." An unnamed physician had suggested roentgen ray treatments, and Friedlander reported the first case of sarcoma of the kidney (Wilms' tumor) treated by radiotherapy. [13] "Treatments were given with the Coolidge tube. Three areas, front, back and side of the tumor, were covered at each treatment, except for the first and second, when one and two areas, respectively, were treated." Treatments were given at intervals of about a week. The dosage varied from 10 to 50 Ma. sec and consisted of 20 treatments between October, 1915, and March, 1916. By the end of the seventh treatment, the child's tumor had decreased markedly and the child had gained several pounds, looked rosy and well and played like an apparently normal child. But in March, 1916, he became listless and apathetic. The tumor had regrown, and the child died following a bout with measles. Necropsy showed a sarcoma of the left kidney with metastases to both lungs and liver.

A review of the literature from the early 1900s to the mid-1930s reveals relatively little progress in treatment of this entity. There were numerous case reports describing the symptoms and therapy, which included surgery and x-ray therapy. [14-17] In 1936, Priestley and Schulte reported on the results of nephrectomy in 39 patients with Wilms' tumor; 6 lived 5 years or more following operation, a survival rate of approximately 15%. [18] Priestley found that preliminary irradiation followed by nephrectomy and, subsequently, postoperative irradiation resulted in the best prognosis. In 1941, Ladd and White[19] described a decreasing mortality rate in Wilms' tumor, from 23% of 30 patients treated from 1914 to 1932 to 3% of patients treated between 1932 and 1941. This impressive result may have been due in part to their decision that the operative technique be performed as soon as the probable diagnosis was made. They were the first to suggest that nephrectomies could be performed in children with minimal morbidity and mortality. Ladd's survival rate was 40% of children treated between 1932 and 1941.

In 1898, William Coley attempted pharmacologic treatment of a renal tumor by administering toxins preoperatively to a 5-year-old child. [20] The child was operated upon and died within a year of surgery. Coley's attempt represents the first trial of systemic agents for this entity. It was not until the mid-1950s that the first specific chemotherapeutic agent for Wilms' tumor was described, when Farber reported that actinomycin D produced tumor regression. [21] In 1963, Sutow et al. showed that vincristine produced significant regression of measurable disease in 8 out of 13 children with disseminated Wilms' tumor.[22] Sutow and his colleagues also showed that the increased use of chemotherapy with actinomycin D and vincristine caused further improvement in the survival rate of children with this tumor.[23] By the late 1960s patients with Wilms' tumor were usually treated with surgery, radiotherapy, and at least two active chemotherapeutic agents. Currently, a cooperative effort by clinicians throughout the country, the National Wilms' Tumor Study Group, is evaluating newer concepts in therapy. These will be described in this monograph. It seems safe to predict that by the end of this decade children with Wilms' tumor, when diagnosed and treated early, will be uniformly cured.

ACKNOWLEDGMENT

The author is grateful to Mr. E. H. Smith for assistance in library research.

REFERENCES

1. Wilms, M.: *Die Mischgeschwülste der Nieren*, Leipzig, Arthur Georgi, 1899, pp. 1–90.
2. Rance, T. F.: Case of fungus haematodes of the kidnies. *Med. Phys. J.* 32:19–25, 1814.
3. Gairdner, E.: Case of fungus haematodes in the kidneys. *Edinb. Med. Surg. J.* 29:312–315, 1828.
4. Van der Byl, F.: Cancerous growth of the kidney, weighing 31 pounds. *Lancet* 2:309, 1856.
5. Annotations: Extirpation of the kidney. *Lancet* 1:889, 1877.
6. Thomasson, B., and Ravitch, M. M.: Wilms' tumor. *Urol. Surv.* 11:83–100, 2:83–99, 1961.
7. Eberth, C. J.: Myoma sarcomatodes renum. *Virchow's Arch. Pathol. Anat. Physiol.* 518–520, 1872.
8. Cohnheim, J.: Congenitales, quergestreiftes Muskelsarkom der Nieren. *Virchow's Arch. Pathol. Anat. Physiol.* 64–69, 1875.
9. Osler, W.: Two cases of striated myo-sarcoma of the kidney. *J. Anat. Physiol.* 14:229–233, 1879.
10. Kocher, T., and Langhans, T.: Eine Nephrotomie wegen Nierensarkom. Zur Histologie des Nierenkrebses. *Dtsch. Z. Chir.* 9:312–328, 1878.
11. Döderlein, A., and Birch-Hirschfeld, F. V.: Embryonale Drüsengeschwulst der Nierengegend im Kindesalter. *Centralbl. Kr. Harn. Sexual-organe*, 5:3–29, 1894.
12. Israel, J.: Erfahrungen über Nierenchirurgie. *Arch. Klin. Chir.* 47:302–463, 1894.
13. Friedlander, A.: Sarcoma of the kidney treated by the roentgen ray. *Am. J. Dis. Child.* 12:328–330, 1916.
14. Foster, E., and Mendilaharzu, J. R.: Embryonal nephrosarcoma in infant. *JAMA* 86:809, 1926.
15. White, W. C.: Wilms' mixed tumor of the kidney. *Ann. Surg.* 9:139–143, 1931.
16. Kretschmer, H. L., and Hibbs, W. G.: Mixed tumors of the kidney in infancy and childhood. *Surg. Gynecol. Obstet.* 52:1–24, 1931.

17. Geschickter, C. F., and Widenhorn, H.: Nephrogenic tumors. *Am. J. Cancer* **22**:620–658, 1934.

18. Priestley, J. T., and Schulte, T. L.: The treatment of Wilms' tumor. *Urology* **47**:7–10, 1942.

19. Ladd, W. E., and White, R. R.: Embryoma of the kidney (Wilms' tumor). *JAMA* **117**:1859–1863, 1941.

20. Coley, W. B.: Wilms' tumor. *Am. J. Surg.* **29**:463–464, 1935.

21. Farber, S., Toch, R., Sears, E. M., and Pinkel, D.: Advances in chemotherapy of cancer in man. In Greenstein, J. P., and Haddow, A. (Eds.): *Advances in Cancer Research*, Vol. 4, Academic Press, New York, 1956, pp. 1–71.

22. Sutow, W., Thurman, W. G., and Windmiller, J.: Vincristine (leurocristine) sulfate in the treatment of children with metastatic Wilms' tumor. *Pediatrics* **32**:880–887, 1963.

23. Sutow, W., Gehan, E., Heyn, R., et al.: Comparison of survival curves, 1956 versus 1962; in children with Wilms' tumor and neuroblastoma; report of the subcommittee on childhood solid tumors, solid tumor task force National Cancer Institute. *Pediatrics* **45**:800–811, 1970.

CHAPTER TWO

Clinical and Biochemical Manifestations of Wilms' Tumor

PHILLIP HOLLAND, M.D.

Professor of Pediatrics
School of Medicine
University of Kentucky
Lexington, Kentucky

CONTENTS

Improvement in the outcome of patients with Wilms' tumor has increased steadily over the past two decades. An increased survival rate is largely dependent on early detection of the tumor by the general practitioner or pediatrician and the subsequent coordinated efforts of the surgeon, pathologist, radiotherapist, and chemotherapist. Improved preoperative management, precise initial determination of the extent of the disease, and detailed clinical evaluation of the patient following primary therapy are important. Detection of Wilms' tumor at the earliest time possible is essential since the extent of disease at surgery is one of the most important factors affecting the outcome.

This chapter includes a review of the classic clinical manifestations in Wilms' tumor and a survey of congenital anomalies whose presence is associated with an increased risk of developing Wilms' tumor. In addition, we review evidence regarding the capacity of Wilms' tumor for secretion of renin, erythropoietin, and an abnormal protein-polysaccharide complex. Knowledge of these factors may assist in early diagnosis of Wilms' tumor.

CLINICAL MANIFESTATIONS

Wilms' tumor is found in the newborn and in the elderly. The peak incidence of Wilms' tumor occurs between the second and third year of life.[1-3] Seventy-eight percent of children are less than 5 years of age at the time of diagnosis of Wilms' tumor.[1,2,4-6] The male to female ratio is 1.2:1.[1-5] Wilms' tumor involves the left kidney in 55% of patients.[1-3,5]

The most common presenting manifestation of Wilms' tumor is a palpable abdominal mass and/or an enlarging abdomen. The presence of the abdominal mass is detected more frequently by parents than by physicians.[1,2] Wilms' tumor is usually a firm, smooth, nontender mass in one of the upper abdominal quadrants and is palpable in the flank but seldom across the midline.[2] Findings on physical examination of the abdomen in each individual are related to the site of tumor origin in the kidney, duration of tumor growth, presence or absence of local extension, and intrarenal necrosis and hemorrhage. A review of additional initial manifestations in 714 infants and children with Wilms' tumor is as follows: Abdominal pain was present in 29% of patients, hematuria in 24%, and fever of undetermined origin in approximately 10%.[1-6] Flank pain occurred in 12 out of 49 cases in one series.[6] Vague symptoms of anorexia, vomiting, and malaise were observed in about 5% of patients. Although hypertension is present in some patients with Wilms' tumor, the incidence is unknown, being reported in as many as 50% in one series,[2] and in less than 5% of 119 patients in two other series.[1,6] The relationship of severe hypertension and increased renin activity with Wilms' tumor will be discussed later. Unusual initial manifestations have included intraperitoneal rupture of Wilms' tumor,[7] cough and pleural pain secondary to pulmonary metastasis,[8] and polycythemia.[9]

Plain roentgenograms of the abdomen may show a mass of increased density displacing the intestines toward the opposite side. Pyelograms are essential to demonstrate the relationship of the tumor to the involved kidney and to evaluate the excretory function of the opposite kidney. Pyelograms of the involved kidney vary greatly and displacement, deformity, distention, or obliteration of the renal pelvis may be present (Figure 1). Arteriography may also provide useful findings (Figure 2).

An abdominal mass of renal origin in the newborn period suggests the presence of hydronephrosis, cystic dysplasia, polycystic disease, mesenchymal hamartoma, or Wilms' tumor. Fetal renal hamartomas[10] (congenital mesoblastic nephromas,[11] "congenital Wilms' tumor," or leiomyoma[12]) are to be distinguished from true Wilms' tumor which is exceedingly rare in the newborn. The microscopic pathology of a fetal renal hamartoma is distinctive and, in all but one unusual case[13] out of the more than 50 cases reported, a benign course without metastasis or local recurrence followed complete excision.[10] Chemotherapy and radiation therapy are of no value and should be avoided because of their potentially harmful effects.

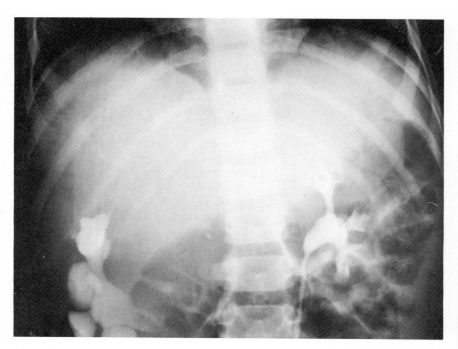

Figure 1. Preoperative IVP showing marked dilatation and distortion of the calical system and inferiolateral displacement of the right kidney. (Courtesy of Dr. Frank Bagnasco.)

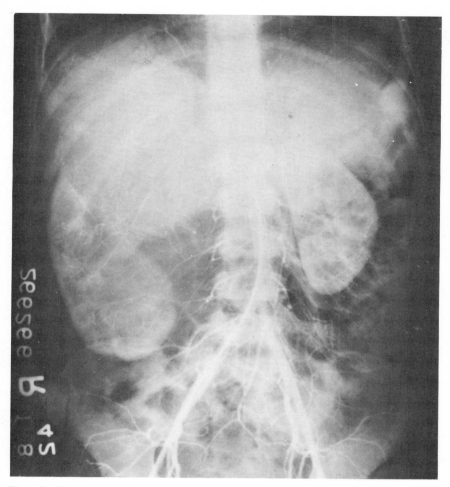

Figure 2. Same patient as Figure 1. Flush aortography and selective right renal angiogram demonstrates a huge mass occupying the upper pole and middle pole of the right kidney, which appears intrarenal as evidenced by distinct beaking. There is minimal to moderate vascularity. Early draining veins are seen. The impression was intrarenal mass occupying the middle and upper pole, displacing the aorta, superior mesenteric artery as well as the liver. This finding is consistent with a Wilms' tumor. (Courtesy of Dr. John Maitem.)

Bilateral Involvement

When embryonal cells from one of paired organs undergo neoplastic transformation, the potential risk for the same cell type in the opposite organ to develop malignancy may be increased. The incidence of bilateral Wilms' tumor has been as high as 10% in one series of 130 patients;[14] the incidence obtained from reviewing several additional series is less. In 3840 cases of Wilms' tumor, bilaterality was recorded in 128 for an incidence of 3.3%.[1,4-6,14-24] Whether bilateral involvement is predominantly the result of separate primary lesions or of metastatic disease is unknown. Recognition of the possibility of bilateral renal involvement in any patient with Wilms' tumor is of prime importance at surgery and also in the year following nephrectomy. If the opposite kidney is affected, appropriate surgical, radiotherapeutic, and chemotherapeutic measures should be instituted at the earliest time possible. (See chapter 9.)

PATTERNS OF METASTASIS AND TUMOR GROWTH

Wilms' tumor may extend through the kidney capsule, invade intrarenal vessels, the renal vein, and inferior vena cava, or spread by the lymphatics to adjacent and distant lymphoid tissue. Direct extension through the capsule is more frequent than distant metastasis.[3,25] Metastatic disease was present at initial diagnosis of Wilms' tumor in 22% of patients, namely, in 253 out of 1102 patients of all ages compiled from six large series.[1-3,5,26,27] The more common sites of metastasis are lung, liver, and lymph nodes; the less common sites are omentum, pleura, skeleton, bone marrow, brain, parotid gland, adrenal gland, pancreas, and tonsils.[1-3,5,26-29] The lung far exceeds the liver as the most frequent site of distant metastasis at the time of diagnosis and following initial therapy. The rounded, nodular pulmonary lesions of Wilms' tumor are variable in size and rarely produce obstructive atelectasis.[30] Skeletal lesions due to Wilms' tumor are uncommon. When present, the lytic lesions most frequently involve the dorsal spine, but have been observed in the skull, ileum, scapula, zygoma, femur, and tibia.[25,29] Rarely, metastatic clumps of Wilms' tumor cells have been demonstrated in a bone marrow aspirate.[29]

Hematologic and serologic abnormalities may be present in children with disseminated Wilms' tumor. Routine initial diagnostic laboratory evaluation includes a complete blood count, platelet count, erythrocyte sedimentation rate, blood urea nitrogen, serum electrolytes and uric acid, hepatic enzymes, alkaline phosphatase, and serum immunoelectrophoretic analysis. A screening coagulogram, including prothrombin time, partial thromboplastin time, and plasma fibrinogen level should also be done. An increased erythrocyte sedimentation rate and serum haptoglobin level (acute phase reactants), elevated serum uric acid, hepatic enzymes, alkaline phosphatase, and blood coagulation abnormalities may be present in patients with disseminated Wilms' tumor.[25]

Rough estimates of the median cell population doubling time in human Wilms' tumor have been obtained employing intravenous colchimide preoperatively and counting cells arrested in metaphase in the removed tumor.[31] A median potential cell population doubling time of 188 hours (7.8 days) was found in Wilms' tumor as compared to 100 hours (4.2 days) in neuroblastoma. Using serial radiographic measurements of the growth of Wilms' tumor pulmonary metastasis, a median value of 20 days was obtained for the overall tumor volume doubling time. From the population doubling time and overall volume doubling time, a speculative analysis was made in one Wilms' tumor which suggested that cells are produced at a rate of at least 5/1000 tumor cells/hr, of which at least 3 are lost from the proliferating pool by necrosis, differentiation, or emigration. These preliminary estimates of Wilms' tumor growth are of interest and the methods outlined serve as additional tools for further studies comparing growth rates in Wilms' tumor and other solid tumors of infancy and childhood. The clinical observation of rapid growth following onset of a Wilms' tumor has been documented.[32]

ASSOCIATED CONGENITAL ANOMALIES

Wilms' tumor is an example of the increasingly recognized association of childhood oncogenesis and teratogenesis. Wilms' tumor is linked with nonfamilial aniridia, hemihypertrophy, the Beckwith-Wiedemann syndrome, ambiguous genitalia with and without focal glomerular renal disease, and possibly with hamartomas.

Aniridia

Miller et al.[33] originally focused attention on the association of Wilms' tumor with aniridia (bilateral absence or hypoplasia of the iris) (Figure 3). Over the past decade at least 28 cases of Wilms' tumor associated with nonfamilial aniridia, cataracts, central nervous system involvement, growth retardation, and anomalies of the genitourinary tract and ear have been documented.[33-46] A summary of the clinical manifestations of the nonfamilial aniridia–Wilms' tumor syndrome is shown in Table 1.

Aniridia occurs in the general population with an incidence of 1:50,000.[47] Nonfamilial aniridia occurs in approximately 1 in 70 children with Wilms' tumor.[33] Familial aniridia is generally inherited as an autosomal dominant gene with high penetrance[38] and is associated with other ocular anomalies but rarely with nonocular congenital defects or Wilms' tumor.

Hemihypertrophy

Congenital hemihypertrophy is associated with Wilms' tumor, hepatocellular and adrenocortical neoplasia,[33] neurofibromatosis,[48] and Silvers' syndrome.[49] The

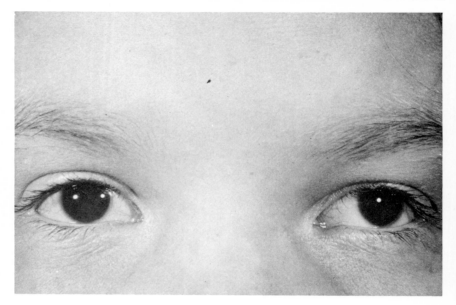

Figure 3.   Aniridia (absence of the iris) in a child with Wilms' tumor.

incidence of hemihypertrophy (Figure 4) has been reported as 1:14,300 births followed until 6 years of age.[50] In a series of 225 children with Wilms' tumor (1:32 incidence)[51] 7 patients with hemihypertrophy were reported. Twenty-seven cases of Wilms' tumor and congenital hemihypertrophy have been recorded;[51,52] of these 20 were females (a 1:2.8 male to female ratio), in contrast to the 1.2:1 male to female ratio observed in Wilms' tumor or hemihypertrophy alone (Figure 2).

Beckwith-Wiedemann Syndrome

The Beckwith-Wiedemann syndrome[53,54] consists of hyperplastic fetal visceromegaly involving the kidney, adrenal cortex, pancreas, gonads, and liver with macroglossia, omphalocele, hemihypertrophy, microcephaly, mental retardation and postnatal somatic gigantism. This syndrome is associated with an increased incidence of neoplastic transformation involving the kidney, adrenal cortex, gonads, and liver. Of 34 cases of the Beckwith-Wiedemann syndrome tabulated by Reddy et al.[55] Wilms' tumor was present in 3, adrenal carcinoma in 3, and gonadoblastoma and hepatoblastoma in 1 case each. Hemihypertrophy was present in 3 of the patients with Beckwith-Wiedemann syndrome and intraabdominal malignancy.[56-58]

Table 1. Associated Anomalies in 28 Patients With Nonfamilial Bilateral Aniridia–Wilms' Tumor Syndrome[33-46]

Associated Anomalies	Incidence (%)

Ocular anomalies
    Cataract
    Glaucoma
	78

Central nervous system involvement
    Mental retardation
    Microcephaly
    Craniofacial dysmorphism
	71

External ear anomalies Deformed pinna	35
Growth retardation	28
Reproductive system anomalies Cryptorchidism	28

Urinary Tract Anomalies
    Hypospadias
    Horseshoe kidney
	21

Mean age	1 yr, 10 mos.

Sexual Ambiguity

The association of congenital renal anomalies with reproductive system anomalies and the association of sexual ambiguity and gonadal neoplasm is well documented.[59] The association of Wilms' tumor with urinary tract anomalies, cryptorchidism, and aniridia has been outlined previously. The occurrence of Wilms' tumor in patients with pseudohermaphroditism has been reported less frequently.[35,59-63] A summary of 7 known patients with pseudohermaphroditism and Wilms' tumor is shown in Table 2; 5 out of 7 were males by buccal smear or leukocyte karyotype, and hypertension was also present in 5 out of 7. Focal glomerular disease with fatal renal failure was present in 3 children with Wilms' tumor and pseudohermaphroditism.[59,63]

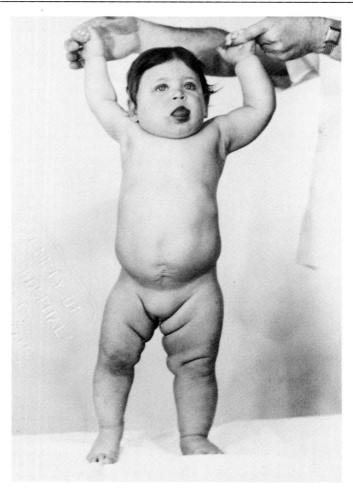

Figure 4.   A child from whom a Wilms' tumor was removed showing crossed hemihypertrophy. The left extremities and the right side of the face are involved. (Courtesy of Dr. Frank Wilson and the *Journal of Bone and Joint Surgery.*[56])

The linkage of Wilms' tumor with the previously outlined congenital anomalies suggests that this neoplasm may be induced by one or more agents with oncogenic as well as teratogenic properties.[64] Recognition and evaluation by the pediatrician, ophthalmologist, neurologist, and surgeon of patients who are at high risk for the development of Wilms' tumor is most important.

Table 2. Clinical Summary of Reported Cases of Wilms' Tumor and Sexual Ambiguity

Patient	Age at Diagnosis of Tumor (Yr/Mo)	Pseudo-hermaphrodite	Sex Determination	Focal Glomerular Disease	Hypertension	Age at Death (yr/mo.)	Cause	Author
1	—	Male	—	Absent	—	1/6	—	Raubitschek[60]
2	1/11–left 2/6–right	Male	Immature testis histologically	Absent	Present	2/1	Bilateral Wilms' tumor	Stump and Gannett[61]
3	3/1	Agonadism	Chromatin negative	Absent	Present	3/10	Metastatic disease	Angstrom[62]
4	2/1	Male	46,XY	—	—	—	—	DiGeorge and Harley[35]
5	0/3	Male	46,XX/XY Mosaic	Present	Present	1/3	Renal failure	Denys et al.[63]
6	1/9	Male	Chromatin negative	Present	Present	7/6	Renal failure	Drash et al.[59]
7	3/6	Male	46,XY	Present	Present	3/10	Renal failure	Drash et al.[59]

Other Reported Disorders

Hamartomas (pigmented nevi and internal hemangiomas) were observed in 8 of 437 cases of Wilms' tumor.[33] Isolated cases of Wilms' tumor with cardiac fibromatous hamartoma,[55] adrenocortical adenoma,[65] and congenital lipoma[42] have also been recorded. Whether the association of Wilms' tumor and hamartoma in these cases exceeds normal expectations is unknown.

Chromosome analyses have been structurally and numerically normal in most patients with Wilms' tumor.[66] Isolated examples of Wilms' tumor and chromosome aberrations include 45,XO Turner's syndrome,[66] 18-trisomy syndrome,[67] elongated arms of number 16 chromosome[51] and a mosaic 46XX/XY.[63]

HYPERTENSION, RENIN ACTIVITY, AND RENAL TUMORS

The true incidence of mild to moderate hypertension in infants and children with Wilms' tumor is unknown. This lack of knowledge is partly due to lack of standard conditions for measuring blood pressures that has resulted in ill-defined normal values at various age periods. Malignant hypertension in Wilms' tumor is uncommon. Only 30 cases of Wilms' tumor and extreme hypertension were documented between 1937 and 1965.[68-76] Of the patients who underwent surgery, 67% were relieved of hypertension in these early reports. A fall in blood pressure following removal of a Wilms' tumor suggested that the hypertension was either the result of compression of the renal artery by the tumor or that a pressor substance was produced by the neoplasm.[68] Recurring hypertension concomitant with the development of metastatic lesions and subsequent return to normotensive levels following radiation therapy of the metastasis further suggested excessive production of a pressor substance such as renin by the tumor.[71]

Elevated tumor renin was first documented in a patient with hypertension and a hemangiopericytoma arising from the renal juxtaglomerular apparatus by Robertson et al.[77] in 1967. Shortly thereafter, Mitchell et al.[78] and Spergel et al.[79] reported elevated plasma renin levels which returned to normal following removal of the affected kidney in two infants with Wilms' tumor and severe hypertension. Voute et al.[80] assayed plasma renin activity pre- and postoperatively in 5 additional children with Wilms' tumor in whom only a moderate elevation of blood pressure was present. A significant decrease in plasma renin activity was observed postoperatively in each patient. Recently, Ganguly et al.[81] reported a markedly elevated renin level in a Wilms' tumor extract in contrast to a negligible renin level in normal kidney cortex adjacent to the tumor. The elevated plasma renin activity returned to normal postoperatively. A summary of the patients with Wilms' tumor and increased renin activity is shown in Table 3. These data provide further evidence that neoplastic cells in a Wilms' tumor may secrete excessive amounts of

Table 3. Comparison of Clinical and Laboratory Data in Wilms' and Renal Juxtaglomerular Cell Tumors With Increased Renin Activity

Case	Age (Yr/Mo)	Blood Pressure (mmHg) Preop	Blood Pressure (mmHg) Postop	Serum Potassium Level Preop (mEq/1)	Peripheral Plasma Renin Activity Preop	Peripheral Plasma Renin Activity Postop	Renal Vein Renin Activity of Involved Kidney	Renal Tumor Renin	Aldosterone Excretion	Reference
				Wilms' Tumor and Increased Renin Activity						
1	0/5	210/160	225/125	2.7	↑	→	—	—	—	79
2	1/11	260/200	75/50	2.8	↑	Normal	—	↑	—	78
3	1/8	105/65	DEATH	—	↑	—	—	—	—	80
4	1/10	105/65	100/60	—	↑	Normal	—	—	—	
5	5/1	128/80	110/70	—	↑	Normal	—	—	—	
6	5/5	135/95	—	—	↑	—	—	—	—	
7	3/11	120/90	110/60	—	↑	Normal	—	—	—	
8	2/7	120/80	105/50	—	↑	—	—	—	—	
9	6/2	135/105	100/60	—	↑	Normal	—	—	—	
10	1/8	110/90	100/50	—	↑	Normal	—	—	—	
11	1/6	160/120	140/90	—	↑	↑	—	—	—	82
12	4/9	200/140	125/80	3.7	↑	Normal	Normal*	↑	↑	81
Mean (3/1)										
				Juxtaglomerular Cell Tumor and Increased Renin Activity						
1	16	250/150	145/90	3.2	—	—	—	↑	—	77
2	23	186/110	Normal	3.4	↑	Normal	—		↑	84
3	37	225/145	115/76	3.0	↑	Normal	—	↑	Normal	85
4	13	190/160	125/70	2.6	↑	Normal	↑	↑	—	83
5	18	200/128	124/86	3.5	↑	Normal	↑	↑	↑	86
6	24	190/130	130/90	3.9	↑	Normal	↑	↑	Normal	87
Mean, (22/0)										

*Patient had received chemotherapy prior to renal vein renin determination.

21

renin and that increased renin production in an involved kidney may not be the result of renal arterial channel compression by the tumor mass (i.e., Goldblatt kidney).

A distinct syndrome of severe hypertension, secondary aldosteronism with hypokalemia, increased plasma renin activity, and a benign tumor of the renal juxtaglomerular apparatus has been identified in young adults (mean age, 23 years).[77,83-87] Presenting manifestations include headache, visual difficulties, dizziness (probably due to hypertension), intermittent muscular weakness (due to hypokalemia), and polyuria (due to kaliopenic nephropathy). Excessive amounts of renin were found in the renal vein blood from the tumor-containing kidney as well as in the excised tumor; adjacent normal kidney tissue contained normal amounts of renin. Conn et al.[86] recently documented in vitro release of renin from explants of the tumor grown in tissue culture; they also showed granular cytoplasmic immunofluorescence in the original tumor cells and in cultured tumor cells when reacted with antihuman renin antibodies. A summary of the patients with documented renin-secreting juxtaglomerular cell tumors is shown in Table 3 for comparison with Wilms' tumor patients. In all of the patients with juxtaglomerular cell tumors blood pressure rapidly returned to normal following removal of the tumor.

ERYTHROPOIETIN ACTIVITY AND WILMS' TUMOR

Polycythemia, primarily involving erythropoiesis, is associated with a variety of cystic and neoplastic lesions of the kidney. Thurman et al.[9] originally reported a patient with Wilms' tumor and polycythemia (hemoglobin 18.2 gm%) in whom increased erythropoietin activity was present in the plasma and in homogenized tumor tissue removed from a pulmonary metastasis. Shalet et al.[88] found a significant amount of erythropoietin in a primary Wilms' tumor from a 20-month-old patient with polycythemia. Murphy et al.[89-90] investigated the correlation of plasma erythropoietin with the clinical and surgical course of patients with Wilms' tumor and with a variety of other spontaneous and experimentally induced renal lesions. None of the patients with Wilms' tumor had an elevated hematocrit. Of 8 patients with Wilms' tumor had elevated plasma erythropoietin levels preoperatively and normal plasma erythropoietin levels were present in all 4 patients studied postoperatively. Recurrence of Wilms' tumor was associated with recurrence of elevated erythropoietin levels. These observations suggested that plasma erythropoietin assay might be helpful in the serial evaluation of children with Wilms' tumor, to monitor the relative success of therapy.

Follow-up data in this series and additional patients with Wilms' tumor have recently been reviewed by Kenny et al.[91] and by Murphy et al.[92] Twenty-five patients were studied for a minimum of 24 months postnephrectomy or until death. The following postnephrectomy observations were made: (a) An elevation of plasma erythropoietin was not observed in the absence of known metastatic disease (greater than 96% correlation). (b) Plasma erythropoientin was elevated in all patients with known clinically active metastatic disease (100%). (c) When metastatic disease was treated successfully, an elevation of plasma erythropoietin was sustained for several months but subsequently returned to normal. These studies provide additional evidence that serial plasma erythropoietin assay is a valuable aid in the clinical evaluation of patients with Wilms' tumor.

Increased erythropoietin activity has also been documented in patients with renal cell carcinoma,[90,93-95] renal adenoma,[93] renal cysts,[90,96,97] hydronephrosis,[90,97,98] cerebellar hemangioblastoma,[90,97,99] pheochromocytoma,[100] uterine fibromyoma,[101] and hepatocellular carcinoma.[93,102,103] The regulatory mechanisms of erythropoietin production and utilization in patients with Wilms' tumor and other benign and malignant disorders of the kidney have been reviewed recently.[104,105]

ABNORMAL SERUM MUCOPOLYSACCHARIDE IN WILMS' TUMOR

The presence of strands of acidophilic background material on Wright's stained blood smears, leukocyte agglutination, erythrocyte rouleau formation, and a white fibrillar precipitate immediately following acidification of the serum in a patient with metastatic Wilms' tumor were first reported by Morse and Nussbaum.[106] A mucopolysaccharide, presumably hyaluronic acid, was identified as the unusual serum component. Powars et al.[107] and Allerton et al.[108] noted this peculiar azurophilic material in blood smears (Figure 5), bone marrow smears, and tumor imprints (Figure 6) prepared with Wright's stain in additional children with metastatic Wilms' tumor. Strongly positive acid mucopolysaccharide staining was present in blood, bone marrow, and tumor imprints. Tumor extracts contained an abnormal electrophoretic component staining as a protein-polysaccharide complex or mucin. Serial determinations of blood mucin were correlated with the clinical status of 6 patients.[109] From these data it appears that the blood concentration of the extracellular mucin increases markedly during periods of aftergrowth of primary metastatic tumor and decreases when the tumor is removed or the growth rate comes under therapeutic control. This mucinous substance was only identified in the peripheral blood and urine in patients whose tumor extended beyond the capsule, that is, Stage II, III, or IV. However, it was present in all tumor specimens examined, regardless of the clinical staging of the tumor.

Further characterization and quantitative analysis of the mucopolysaccharide complex may allow this serum determination to be helpful in initial diagnosis, staging of Wilms' tumor, and detection of metastases in the postoperative patient.

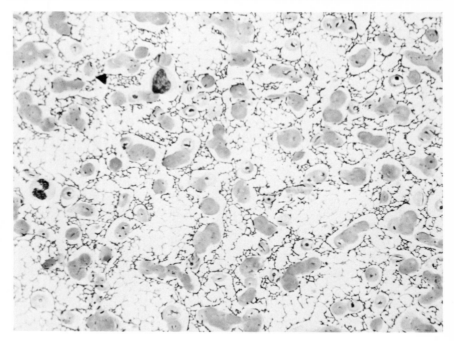

Figure 5.   Peripheral blood smear, stained with Wright's stain, of a patient with extensive metastatic Wilms' tumor and massive amounts of azurophilic staining material. (Courtesy of Dr. Darleen Powars and Dr. Samuel Allerton.)

CONCLUSIONS

Careful palpation of the abdomen is an integral part of each routine physical examination in infancy and childhood. The pediatrician or general practitioner may perform thousands of abdominal examinations, yet may rarely palpate a small, silent Wilms' tumor. This discovery, in even a single patient, is ample reward for the many hours spent in the diligent examination of normal infants and children. Abdominal pain, flank pain, hematuria, unexplained fever, anorexia, and vomiting are the more frequently encountered symptoms accompanying the presence of an abdominal mass or enlarging abdomen due to Wilms' tumor. A suspicion of Wilms' tumor should be aroused when patients are encountered who are at increased risk because of the following isolated congenital anomalies or syndromes: (a) nonfamilial aniridia, cataracts, mental retardation, external ear deformity, cryptorchidism, and hypospadias, (b) isolated hemihypertrophy, (c) hyperplastic fetal visceromegaly, omphalocele, macroglossia, hemihypertrophy,

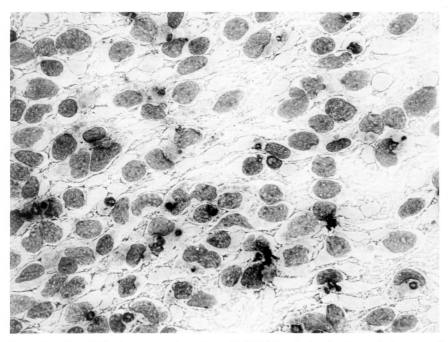

Figure 6.   Direct Wilms' tumor imprint stained with Wright's stain showing the marked amount of mucin in the stroma of the tumor. (Courtesy of Dr. Darleen Powars and Dr. Samuel Allerton.)

microcephaly with mental retardation and postnatal somatic gigantism, and (d) pseudohermaphroditism.

The following recent observations suggest that Wilms' tumor is a secretory neoplasm: (a) Increased plasma and tumor renin activity has been found in patients with Wilms' tumor and hypertension. (b) Increased plasma erythropoietin has been found in patients with Wilms' tumor pre-operatively, and in postoperative patients with known clinically active metastatic disease. Postoperatively and following successful treatment of metastatic disease the plasma erythropoietin levels returned to normal. (c) An abnormal protein-polysaccharide complex has been detected in the serum, urine, and cellfree tumor extracts from patients with Wilms' tumor. Presence of these mucinous components in serial serum samples has correlated with the known clinical status of the patients. Further clinical studies of these Wilms' tumor secretion products may provide sensitive indicators of tumor activity. These determinations may become as important in Wilms' tumor patients as urinary catecholamine excretion is in the diagnosis and subsequent evaluation of patients with neuroblastoma.

REFERENCES

1.   Sullivan, M. P., Hussey, D. H., and Ayala, A. G.: Wilms' tumor. In Sutow, W., Vietti, T. J., and Fernbach, D. (Eds.): *Clinical Pediatric Oncology,* C. V. Mosby Company, St. Louis, 1973, pp. 359–383.

2.   Silva-Sosa, M., and Gonzalex-Cerna, J. L.: Wilms' tumor in children. *Progr. Clin. Cancer* 2:323–337, 1966.

3.   Ledlie, E. M., Mynors, L. S., Draper, G. J., and Gorbach, P. D.: Natural history and treatment of Wilms' tumour: an analysis of 335 cases occurring in England and Wales 1962–66. *Br. Med. J.* 4:195–200, 1970.

4.   Bjelke, E.: Malignant neoplasms of the kidney in children. *Cancer* 17:318–321, 1964.

5.   Westra, P., Kieffer, S. A., and Mosser, D. G.: Wilms' tumor: a summary of 25 years of experience before actinomycin-D. *Am. J. Roentgenol.* 100:214–221, 1967.

6.   Kenny, G. M., Webster, J. H., Sinks, L. M., et al.: Results from treatment of Wilms' tumor at Roswell Park 1927–1968. *J. Surg. Oncol.* 1:49–61, 1969.

7.   Pochedly, C., Waldman, A., and Kenigsberg, K.: Two and one-half year survival of patient with Wilms' tumor. *JAMA* 216:334, 1971.

8.   Dargeon, H.: *Tumors of childhood,* Paul B. Hoeber, New York, 1960, p. 237.

9.   Thurman, W., Grabstald, H., and Lieberman, P.: Elevation of erythropoietin levels in association with Wilms' tumor. *Arch. Intern. Med.* 117:280–283, 1966.

10. Berdon, W. E., Wigger, H. J., and Baker, D. H.: Fetal renal harmatoma—a benign tumor to be distinguished from Wilms' tumor; report of 3 cases. *Am. J. Roentgenol.* 118:18–27, 1973.

11. Bolande, R. P., Brough, A. J., and Izant, R.: Congenital mesoblastic nephroma of infancy; a report of 8 cases and relationship to Wilms' tumor. *Pediatrics* 40:272–278, 1967.

12. McCune, W. R., Galleher, E. P., and Wood, C.: Leiomyoma of the kidney in a newborn infant. *J. Urol.* 91:646–648, 1964.

13. Walker, D., and Richard, G. A.: Fetal hamartoma of the kidney; recurrence and death of patient. *J. Urol.* 110:352–353, 1974.

14. Jagasia, K. H., Thurman, W. G., Pickett, E., and Grabstaldt, H.: Bilateral Wilms' tumors in children. *J. Pediatr.* 65:371–376, 1964.

15. Martin, L. W., and Kleocker, R. J.: Bilateral nephroblastoma (Wilms' tumor). *Pediatrics* 28:101–106, 1961.

16. Scott, L. S.: Bilateral Wilms' tumour. *Br. J. Surg.* 42:513–516, 1954–1955.

17. Rickham, P. P.: Bilateral Wilms' tumour. *Br. J. Surg.* 44:492–495, 1956–1957.

18. Gross, R. E., and Neuhauser, E. B. D.: Treatment of mixed tumors of kidneys in childhood. *Pediatrics* 6:843–852, 1950.

19. Bishop, H. C., and Hope, J. W.: Bilateral Wilms' tumors. *J. Pediatr. Surg.* 1:476–487, 1966.

20. Abeshouse, B. S.: The management of Wilms' tumor as determined by national survey and review of the literature. *J. Urol.* 77:792–813, 1957.

21. Creevy, C. D., and Reiser, M. P.: Wilms' tumor. *Bull. Univ. Minnesota Hosp. Minnesota Med. Found.* 22:292–300, 1951.

22. Ragab, A. H., Vietti, T. J., Crist, W., Perez, C., and McAllister, W.: Bilateral Wilms' tumor. *Cancer* 30:983–988, 1972.

23. Walker, G.: Sarcoma of kidney in children; a critical review of the pathology, symptomatology, prognosis and operative treatment as seen in 145 cases. *Ann. Surg.* 26:529–602, 1897.

24. Holland, P., and Hellebusch, A.: Therapy in Wilms' tumor of childhood. *J. Ky. Med. Assoc.* 68:645–647, 1970.

25. Pochedly, C.: Wilms' tumor I. Clinical features and tumor biology. *N.Y. State J. Med.* 71:1089–1094, 1971.

26. Jereb, B.: Metastases and recurrences in nephroblastoma. *Acta Radiol. Ther. (Stockh.)* 12:289–304, 1973.

27. Sutow, W. W., Gehan, E. A., Heyn, R. M., et al.: Comparison of survival curves, 1956 versus 1962, in children with Wilms' tumor and neuroblastoma. *Pediatrics* 45:800–811, 1970.

28. Movassaghi, N., Leikin, S., and Chandra, R.: Wilms' tumor metastasis to uncommon sites. *J. Pediatr.* 84:416–417, 1974.

29. O'Neill, P., and Pinkel, D.: Wilms' tumor in bone marrow aspirate. *J. Pediatr.* 72:396–398, 1968.

30. Caffey, J.:*Pediatric X-Ray Diagnosis*, 5th ed., Year Book Medical Publishers, Chicago, 1967, pp. 295–296.

31. Aherne, W., and Buck, P.: The potential cell population doubling time in neuroblastoma and nephroblastoma. *Br. J. Cancer* 25:691–696, 1971.

32. Rabinowitz, J. G., and Bagnasco, F. M.: Wilms' tumor demonstrating onset and rapid growth. *J. Urol.* 103:86–88, 1970.

33. Miller, R. W., Fraumeni, J. F., and Manning, M. D.: Association of Wilms' tumor with aniridia, hemihypertrophy and other congenital malformations. *N. Engl. J. Med.* 270:922–927, 1964.

34. Fontana, V. J., Ferrara, A., and Perciaccante, R.: Wilms' tumor and associated anomalies. *Am. J. Dis. Child.* 109:459–461, 1965.

35. DiGeorge, A. M., and Harley, R. D.: The association of aniridia, Wilms' tumor, and genital abnormalities. *Arch. Ophthalmol.* 75:796–798, 1966.

36. Mackintosh, T. F., Girdwood, T. G., Parker, D. J., and Strachan, I. M.: Aniridia and Wilms' tumour (nephroblastoma). *Br. J. Ophthalmol.* 52:846–848, 1968.

37. Flanagan, J. C., and DiGeorge, A. M.: Sporadic aniridia and Wilms' tumor. *Am. J. Ophthalmol.* 67:558–561, 1969.

38. Fraumeni, J. F., and Glass, A. G.: Wilms' tumor and congenital aniridia. *JAMA* 206:825–828, 1968.

39. Brusa, P., and Torricelli, C.: Nefroblastoma di Wilms ed affezioni renali congenite nella casistica dell'I. P.P.A.I. di Milano. *Minerva Pediatr.* 5:457–463, 1953.

40. Schweisguth, O., Campinchi, R., Pivoteav, B., and Lemerle, J.: L'association aniridie —tumeur du rein chez l'enfant; à propos de 4 cas. *Bull. Soc. Ophthalmol. Fr.* 67:1099–1107, 1967.

41. Zimmerman, L. E., and Font, R. L.: Congenital malformations of the eye. Some recent advances in knowledge of the pathogenesis and histopathological characteristics. *JAMA* 196:684–692, 1966.

42. Haicken, B. N., and Miller, D. R.: Simultaneous occurrence of congenital aniridia, hamartoma, and Wilms' tumor. *J. Pediatr.* 78:497–502, 1971.

43. Evans, D. I. K., and Holzel, A.: Wilms'–aniridia syndrome with transient hypo-γ-globulinaemia of infancy. *Arch. Dis. Child.* 48:645–646, 1973.

44. Woodard, J. R., and Levine, M. K.: Nephroblastoma (Wilms' tumor) and congenital aniridia. *J. Urol.* 101:140–143, 1969.

45. Neidhardt, M.: Wilms-tumor und aniridie—ein genetisch fixiertes syndrom. *Klin. Paediatr.* 184:312–317, 1972.

46. Gandhi, R. K., Deshmukh, S. S., and Waingankar, V. S.: Wilms' tumor with aniridia. *J. Pediatr. Surg.* 5:571, 1970.

47. Shaw, M. W., Falls, H. F., and Neel, J. V.: Congenital aniridia. *Am. J. Hum. Genet.* 12:389–415, 1960.

48. Moore, B. H.: Some orthopaedic relationships of neurofibromatosis. *J. Bone Joint Surg.* 23A:109–140, 1941.

49. Silver, H. K.: Asymmetry, short stature, and variations in sexual development. *Am. J. Dis. Child.* 107:495–515, 1964.

50. Leck, I., Record, R. G., McKeown, T., and Edwards, J. H.: The incidence of malformations in Birmingham, England, 1950–1959. *Teratology* 1:263–280, 1968.

51. Fraumeni, J. F., Geiser, C. F., and Manning, M. D.: Wilms' tumor and congenital hemihypertrophy; report of five new cases and review of literature. *Pediatrics* 40:886–899, 1967

52. Boxer, L., and Smith, D.: Wilms' tumor prior to onset of hemihypertrophy, *Am. J. Dis. Child.* 120:564–565, 1970.

53. Beckwith, J. B., Wang, C., Donnell, G. N., et al.: Hyperplastic fetal visceromegaly, with macroglossia, omphalocele, cytomegaly of the adrenal fetal cortex, postnatal somatic gigantism and other abnormalities; a newly recognized syndrome, abstracted (abstract). Meeting of American Pediatric Society, Seattle, June 16–18, 1964.

54. Wiedemann, H. R.: Complexe malformatif familial avec hernie ombilicale et macroglossie, un "syndrome nouveau." *J. Genet. Hum.* 13:223–232, 1964.

55. Reddy, J. K., Schimke, R. N., Chang, C. H. J., et al.: Beckwith-Wiedemann Syndrome. Wilms' tumor, cardiac hamartoma, persistent visceromegaly, and glomeruloneogenesis in a 2-year-old boy. *Arch. Pathol.* 94:523–532, 1972.

56. Wilson, F. C., and Orlin, H.: Crossed congenital hemihypertrophy associated with a Wilms' tumor. Report of a case. *J. Bone Joint Surg.* 47A:1609–1614, 1965.

57. Harwood, J., and O'Flynn, E.: Specimens from a case of right-sided hemihypertrophy associated with pubertas praecox. *Proc. R. Soc. Med.* 28:837–839, 1935.

58. Weinstein, R. L., Kliman, B., Neeman, J., and Cohen, R. B.: Deficient 17–hydroxylation in a corticosterone producing adrenal tumor from an infant with hemihypertrophy and visceromegaly. *J. Clin. Endocrinol. Metab.* 30:457–468, 1970.

59. Drash, A., Sherman, F., Hartmann, W. H., and Blizzard, R. M.: A syndrome of pseudohermaphroditism, Wilms' tumor, hypertension, and degenerative renal disease. *J. Pediatr.* 76:585–593, 1970.

60. Raubitschek, H.: Über eine bösartige nierengeschwulst bei einem kindlichen hermaphroditen. *Fr. Z. Pathol.* 10:206–218, 1912.

61. Stump, T. A., and Ganett, R. A.: Bilateral Wilms' tumor in a male pseudohermaphrodite. *J. Urol.* 72:1146–1152, 1954.

62. Angstrom, T.: Nephroblastoma in a case of agonadism. *Cancer* 18:857–862, 1965.

63. Denys, P., Malvaux, P., Van den Berghe, H., Tanghe, W., and Proesmans, W.: Association d'un syndrome anatomopathologique de pseudohermaphrodisme masculin, d'une tumeur de Wilms, d'une nephropathie parenchymateuse et d'un mosaicisme XX/XY. *Arch. Fr. Pediatr.* 24:729–739, 1967.

64. Miller, R. W.: Relation between cancer and congenital defects: An epidemiological evaluation. *J. Natl. Cancer Inst.* 40:1079–1085, 1968.

65. Reidel, H. A.: Adrenogenital syndrome in a male child due to adrenocortical tumor; report of case with hemihypertrophy and subsequent development of embryoma (Wilms' tumor). *Pediatrics* 10:19–27, 1952.

66. Say, B., Balci, S., and Tuncbilek, E.: 45, XO Turner's syndrome, Wilms' tumor and imperforate anus. *Humangenet.* **12**:348–350, 1971.

67. Geiser, C. F., and Schindler, A. M.: Long survival in a male with 18–trisomy syndrome and Wilms' tumor. *Pediatrics* **44**:111–116, 1969.

68. Bradley, J. E., and Pincoffs M. C.: The association of adeno-myo-sarcoma of the kidney (Wilms' tumor) with arterial hypertension. *Ann. Intern. Med.* **11**:1613–1628, 1938.

69. Daniel, W. E.: The hypertensive factor in Wilms' tumor. *South Med. J.* **32**:1014–1016, 1939.

70. Koons, K. M., and Ruch, M. K.: Hypertension in a 7-year-old girl with Wilms' tumor relieved by nephrectomy. *JAMA* **115**:1097–1098, 1940.

71. Bradley, J. E., and Drake, M. E.: The effect of preoperative roentgenray therapy on arterial hypertension in embryoma (kidney). *J. Pediatr.* **35**:710–714, 1949.

72. Hughes, J. G., Rosenblum, H., and Horn, L. G.: Hypertension in embryoma (Wilms' tumor). *Pediatrics* **3**:201–207, 1949.

73. Silver, H. K.: Wilms' tumor (embryoma of the kidney). *J. Pediatr.* **31**:643–650, 1947.

74. Gooding, C. A., and Raslavicius, P. A.: Arteriographic demonstration of perirenal hematoma and Wilms' tumor in a hypertensive child. *Am. J. Roentgenol.* **93**:467–472, 1965.

75. Case records of the Massachusetts General Hospital. Case 44061. *N. Engl. J. Med.* **258**:289–295, 1958.

76. Pincoffs, M. C., and Bradley, J. E.: The association of adenosarcoma of the kidney (Wilms' tumor) with arterial hypertension. *Trans. Assoc. Am. Physicians* **52**:320–325, 1937.

77. Robertson, P. W., Klidjian, A., Harding, L. K., and Walters, G.: Hypertension due to a renin-secreting renal tumour. *Am. J. Med.* **43**:963–976, 1967.

78. Mitchell, J. D., Baxter, T. J., Blair-West, J. R., and McCredie, D. A.: Renin levels in nephroblastoma (Wilms' tumour); report of a renin secreting tumour. *Arch. Dis. Child.* **45**:376–384, 1970.

79. Spergel, G., Lustik, B., Levy, L. J., and Ertel, N. H.: Studies of hypertension and carbohydrate intolerance associated with Wilms' tumor. *Ann. Intern. Med.* **70**:565–570, 1969.

80. Voute, P. A., van der Meer, J., and Staugaard-Kloosterziel, W.: Plasma renin activity in Wilms' tumour. *Acta Endocrinol. (Kbh)* **67**:197–202, 1971.

81. Ganguly, A., Gribble, J., Tune, B., et al.: Renin-secreting Wilms' tumor with severe hypertension; report of a case and brief review of renin-secreting tumors. *Ann. Intern. Med.* **79**:835–837, 1973.

82. Marosvári, I., Kontor, E., and Kállay, K.: Renin-secreting Wilms' tumour. *Lancet* **1**:1180–1181, 1972.

83. Bonnin, J. M., Hodge, R. L., and Lumbers, E. R.: A renin-secreting renal tumour associated with hypertension. *Aust. N. Z. J. Med.* **2**:178–181, 1972.

84. Kihara, I., Kitamura, S., Hoshino, T., et al.: A hitherto unreported vascular tumor of the kidney; a proposal of "juxtaglomerular cell tumor." *Acta Pathol. Jap.* **18**:197–206, 1968.

85. Eddy, R. L., and Sanchez, S. A.: Renin-secreting renal neoplasm and hypertension with hypokalemia. *Ann. Intern. Med.* **75**:725–729, 1971.

86. Conn, J. W., Cohen, E. L., Lucas, C. P., et al.: Primary reninism; hypertension, hyperreninemia, and secondary aldosteronism due to renin-producing juxtaglomerular cell tumors. *Arch. Intern. Med.* **130**:682–696, 1972.

87. Schambelan, M., Howes, E. L., Stockigt, J. R., et al.: Role of renin and aldosterone in hypertension due to a renin-secreting tumor. *Am. J. Med.* **55**:86–92, 1973.

88. Shalet, M. F., Holder, T. M., and Walters, T. R.: Erythropoietin-producing Wilms' tumor. *J. Pediatr.* **70**:615–617, 1967.

89. Murphy, G. P., Mirand, E. A., Johnston, G. S., et al.: Erythropoietin release associated with Wilms' tumor. 120:26–32, 1967.

90. Murphy, G. P., Mirand, E. A., Johnston, G. S., et al.: Erythropoietin alterations in human genito-urinary disease states; correlation with experimental observations. *J. Urol.* 99:802–810, 1968.

91. Kenny, G. M., Mirand, E. A., Staubitz, W. J., et al.: Erythropoietin levels in Wilms' tumor patients. *J. Urol.* 104:758–761, 1970.

92. Murphy, G. P., Allen, J. E., Staubitz, W. J., et al.: Erythropoietin levels in patients with Wilms' tumor. *N.Y. State J. Med.* 72:487–489, 1972.

93. Donati, R. M., McCarthy, J. M., Lange, R. D., and Gallagher, N. I.: Erythrocythemia and neoplastic tumors. *Ann. Intern. Med.* 58:47–55, 1963.

94. Thorling, E. B., and Ersbak, J.: Erythrocytosis and hypernephroma. *Scand. J. Haematol.* 1:38–46, 1964.

95. Rosenbach, L. M., and Xefteris, E. D.: Erythrocytosis associated with carcinoma of the kidney. *JAMA* 176:136–137, 1961.

96. Rosse, W. F., Waldmann, T. A., and Cohen, P.: Renal cysts, erythropoietin, and polycythemia. *Am. J. Med.* 34:76–81, 1963.

97. Waldmann, T. A.: Polycythemia and cancer. In *Fifth National Conference Proceedings, 1964*, J.B. Lippincott Company, Philadelphia, 1965, pp. 437–443.

98. Lange, R. D., and Gallagher, N. I.: Clinical and experimental observations on the relationship of the kidney to erythropoietin production. In Jacobson, L. O., and Doyle, M. (Eds.): *Erythropoiesis*, Grune and Stratton, New York, 1962, pp. 361–373.

99. Waldmann, T. A., Levin, E. H., and Baldwin, M.: The association of polycythemia with a cerebellar hemangioblastoma. *Am. J. Med.* 31:318–324, 1961.

100. Waldmann, T. A., and Bradley, J. E.: Polycythemia secondary to a pheochromocytoma with production of an erythropoiesis stimulating factor by the tumor. *Proc. Soc. Exp. Biol. Med.* 108:425–427, 1961.

101. Ossias, A. L., Zanjani, E. D., Zalusky, R., et al.: Case report; studies on the mechanism of erythrocytosis associated with a uterine fibromyoma. *Br. J. Haematol.* 25:179–185, 1973.

102. Santer, M. A., Waldmann, T. A., and Fallon, H. J.: Erythrocytosis and hyperlipemia as manifestations of hepatic carcinoma. *Arch. Intern. Med.* 120:735–739, 1967.

103. Lehman, C. J., Erslev, A. J., and Myerson, R. M.: Erythrocytosis associated with hepatocellular carcinoma. *Am. J. Med.* 35:439–442, 1963.

104. Krantz, S. B., and Jacobson, L. O.: *Erythropoietin and the Regulation of Erythropoiesis*, University of Chicago Press, Chicago, 1970, pp. 176–195.

105. Rajaram, S., and Zanjani, E. D.: Increased production of erythropoietin in a child with Wilms' tumor. *Nassau Cty. Med. Cent. Proc.* 1:97–108, 1974.

106. Morse, B. S., and Nussbaum, M.: The detection of hyaluronic acid in the serum and urine of a patient with nephroblastoma. *Am. J. Med.* 42:996–1002, 1967.

107. Powars, D. R., Allerton, S. E., Beierle, J., and Butler, B. B.: Wilms' tumor clinical correlation with circulating mucin in three cases. *Cancer* 29:1597–1605, 1972.

108. Allerton, S. E., Beierle, J. W., Powars, D. R., and Bavetta, L. A.: Abnormal extracellular components in Wilms' tumor. *Cancer Res.* 30:679–683, 1970.

109. Powars, D. R., and Allerton, S. E.: Personal communication, 1975.

CHAPTER THREE

Radiographic, Angiographic, and Radiokinetic Findings in Wilms' Tumors

J.R. COPE, R.D., M.D., M.B.

Consultant Radiologist,
Southport and Ormskirk Hospitals,
Lancashire, England

CONTENTS

INTRODUCTION

The diagnosis of Wilms' tumor is not difficult to make, if it is based on an accurate history and careful physical examination.[1] Management often consists of immediate excretory urography followed by nephrectomy. Urgent therapy, without wasting time on exhaustive investigations, has been considered obligatory.[2] This philosophy was at least partly responsible for an erroneous diagnosis of Wilms' tumor in 32% of 856 cases and for a warning against regarding every abdominal tumor in children under 10 years as a nephroblastoma.[3] The major diagnostic difficulties arise in those patients who present with similar clinical and radiological features but have a disease other than Wilms' tumor. The dangers of preoperative chemotherapy in such patients has been stressed,[4] and nephrectomy and radiotherapy have been reported in patients who did not have a neoplasm.[5]

In the past, it has been claimed that Wilms' tumor cannot be distinguished from other tumors, cysts, or multicystic disease.[6] Although reasonable doubt often exists in 20 to 30% of such cases after urography, they can and should be evaluated further especially if preoperative chemotherapy or radiotherapy is contemplated, when a correct diagnosis will be achieved in all but a few cases.[7] Since these tumors may have been present for months or years many older clinical maxims are no longer valid.[8] These include: "the sun should not set on a child with an abdominal mass," and "the diagnosis of an abdominal mass in a child consists of an excretory urogram, a chest film and a laparotomy." It seems unlikely that a short delay, during which further investigations are performed, will worsen the prognosis.[9]

It should be borne in mind that although more than 50% of abdominal masses in the neonatal period are likely to be renal,[10] hydronephrosis and varieties of cystic disease will account for a large proportion of these and Wilms' tumors are relatively uncommon.[5] Over the whole period of infancy, congenital multicystic kidney is the most common abdominal mass lesion.[11]

In practice, the differentiation between Wilms' tumor and neuroblastoma constitutes the most frequent and important diagnostic problem. Both tumors are common, rapidly growing, upper abdominal neoplasms occurring in the same age group.

RADIOLOGIC FINDINGS

These have been fully described elsewhere.[12] The radiologic features of some of the more important conditions that figure in the differential diagnosis of Wilms' tumor are summarized in Table 1.

Table 1. Radiographic Differentiation of Wilms' Tumor From Other Diseases Affecting the Kidneys

Disease	Survey Films	Urogram	Angiography
Congenital multicystic kidney	Flank mass displacing bowel gas common. Calcification only in adult cases. No function.	Absent or atretic proximal ureter Pseudodiverticula in distal ureter are common. Absent pelvicaliceal system.	Absent or markedly hypoplastic renal artery with no collaterals.
Congenital unilateral hydronephrosis	Well-defined enlarged renal outline. Bulging of the flank is rare, but psoas shadow is usually lost. Calcification never present. Function may be absent but late appearance of rounded "pools" more common. Perhaps "crescent sign."	Dilated pelvis and calices. Ureter of normal caliber distal to site of obstruction.	Normal renal artery. Stretching of interlobar branches. Delayed nephrogram.
Renal hamartoma	Tuberous sclerosis may be present. Calcification: whorled, linear or "popcorn." Translucencies due to fat. Defects in nephrograms.		Characteristic "beaded" vessels. Cysts or tumors in other areas may be noted with midstream injection.

Renal dysplasia	Kidneys smooth and enlarged. Defects in nephrogram. Stretching of pelvis and calices.	Thin, elongated attenuated vessels, but appearances very similar to those in Wilms' may be found (?). Vessels essentially the same in these two conditions.
Renal cell carcinoma	Rare under 7 years. Amputation of a calix common.	Normal ureter. May be displaced medially in its upper part. Destruction and invasion of pelvis and calices.
Neuroblastoma	Bony metastases common. Bowel gas displacement and bulging of the flank are uncommon and never marked. Calcification is commoner than in Wilms' tumor. Dense, extensive and may be characteristically "speckled," can occur in retroperitoneal nodes. Stretching of upper renal pole with elongation of upper major calix common. Entire kidney may be displaced. Displacements and distortions are essentially extrarenal.	Extrarenal blood supply. More profuse vascularity. If intrarenal, appearances identical with Wilms' tumor may be seen.

Plain Films

These are essential preliminaries to all contrast studies of the urinary tract and may provide important and sometimes diagnostic information. Bulging of the flank (Figure 1), common in nephroblastoma, is seen in nearly 75% of cases. Since it is sometimes difficult to determine its presence, comparison with the normal side may be helpful. A large tumor will also obliterate the normal properitoneal fat line. It is uncommon in neuroblastoma and hydronephrosis. Loss of renal outline accompanies two-thirds of tumors. The soft tissue renal opacity cannot be defined (Figure 1).

Enlargement of the renal outline is seen in one-third of tumors. It is smooth and often massive. An enlarged renal mass is also common in cases of congenital unilateral hydronephrosis, when it is always well defined. Both kidneys may be smoothly enlarged in cases of cystic disease and renal dysplasia. Displacement of bowel gas (Figure 2) is evident in more than half the tumors and implies considerable forward expansion of the kidney. This sign is made more obvious as the vast majority of patients, being infants, have gas delineating their small bowel as well as their stomach and colon. Bowel gas is usually displaced to the opposite flank so that the affected kidney is often free from overlying bowel gas shadows. Upward and downward displacement of bowel gas, leaving only the loin free, results from less marked changes. Bowel gas displacement is infrequent in neuroblastoma and is never marked, but usually occurs in the congenital multicystic kidney.

Loss of the psoas shadow is seen in one-third of cases. It can only be assumed to be present when the contralateral shadow is clearly visible. Normally, both psoas shadows are frequently absent.

Calcification is present in 10 to 15% of cases. Both curvilinear and punctuate opacities may be present, but the calcification is subtle and never dense. In contrast, calcification in neuroblastoma is much commoner and may be characteristically speckled. It is frequently dense and extensive and may also be evident in the retroperitoneal lymph nodes. A renal hamartoma, which may be associated with tuberous sclerosis, may contain either whorled or linear calcification; "popcorn" calcification, as in the pulmonary hamartoma, is characteristic but rarer. A radiolucency, due to its fat content, may also be apparent within the renal outline.

Atypical features, which should arouse doubt about a diagnosis of Wilms' tumor, include: (1) dense or extensive calcification, (2) a well-defined renal outline, (3) no displacement of bowel gas with a large tumor, and (4) no bulging of the flank with a large tumor.

Excretory Urography

This is the major examination in the identification of urinary tract disease. Modern high-dosage techniques should be employed. Although there is rarely any

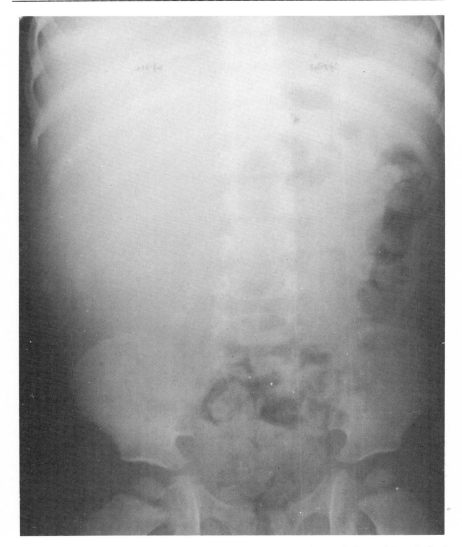

Figure 1. Plain film of the abdomen of a child with Wilms' tumor showing bulging of the right flank and loss of renal outline.

requirement for gaseous distention of the stomach in infants, tomography is virtually routine. Impaired renal function is found in one-fifth of cases. It is present when the involved kidney fails to produce a prompt, dense pyelogram. Total loss of function is extremely rare. Complete nonfunction is characteristic of

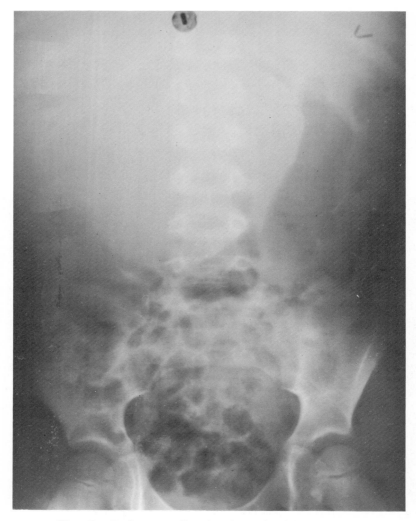

Figure 2.   Displacement of bowel gas by a right-sided Wilms' tumor.

the congenital multicystic kidney. In congenital hydronephrosis, function can again be entirely suppressed but reduced; delayed function is more common.

Displacement of the pelvicaliceal system is seen in approximately two-thirds of tumors. It is frequently the most remarkable single feature (Figure 3A). These displacements can be very marked, the pelvis and calices being pushed away from the tumor mass, usually forward, medially and either upward or downward; the degree of displacement may be such that both collecting systems lie in the same side of the abdomen (Figure 3B). These grossly misplaced calices, which may overlie ribs or bony pelvis, can easily be overlooked and lead to an erroneous conclusion of renal nonfunction. A neuroblastoma may displace the entire kidney, as well as the pelvis and calices, especially laterally and forward. Usually, tomographic cuts will reveal the essential extrarenal nature of this displacement. Although in many varieties of hamartoma and renal dysplasia there is stretching of the pelvis and calices, other signs, such as defects in the nephrogram, will also be present.

Distortion of the pelvicaliceal system is encountered in over 50% of patients.

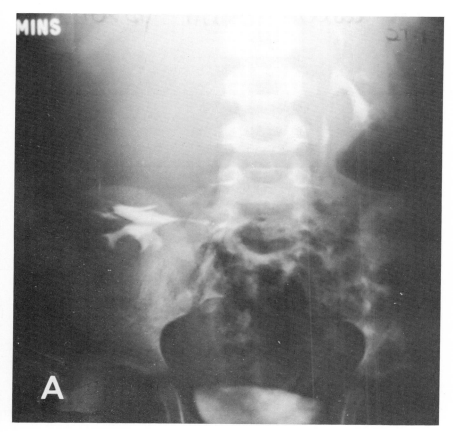

Figure 3. (A) Displacement of the pelvicaliceal system by a Wilms' tumor of the upper pole of the right kidney. (B) Displacement of the pelvicaliceal system by a huge left-sided Wilms' tumor; both collecting systems lie on the same siade of the abdomen.

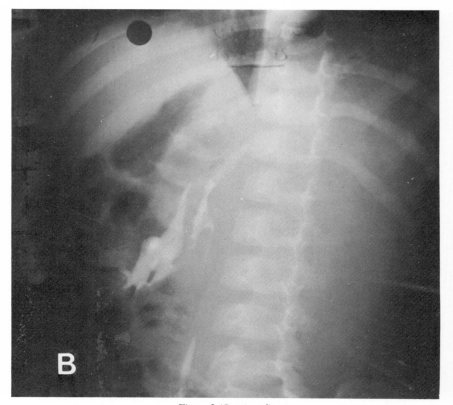

Figure 3 (Continued)

The overall pattern is often bizarre and highly characteristic. Major calices are elongated and are displaced in a curvilinear fashion around the margins of the tumor while minor calices are either bulged in their transverse diameters or are flattened (Figure 4A). Renal cell carcinoma, rare below 7 years of age, has been reported in adolescents and is similar in appearance to Wilms' tumor.[13] A small expanding lesion deforming or amputating a calix, however, is common in carcinoma and is not seen in Wilms' tumor. Involvement of the renal capsule in neuroblastoma can lead to stretching of the upper renal pole with elongation of the upper major calix. Again it is usually clear, especially on tomography, that this distortion is essentially extrinsic. The renal pelvis is intact, albeit displaced (Figure 4B). Unfortunately, a neuroblastoma can occasionaly arise intrarenally when appearances indistinguishable from Wilms' tumor are produced. A proven example is illustrated, showing invasion of the renal pelvis (Figure 4C).

Enlargement of the pelvicaliceal system is encountered in 40% of tumors. It varies from a localized hydrocalycosis (Figure 5A) to dilatation of all the major calices (Figure 5B, ⅝C). Pelvic hydronephrosis is not a feature of Wilms' tumor. Rounded pools of contrast medium, unchanged on prone films, appear late during urography in cases of congenital hydronephrosis (Figure 6). A "crescent" may sometimes be seen, representing a nephrogram in functioning parenchyma which is compressed by a dilated pelvis.[14] The duplex kidney can cause diagnostic difficulties when diseased, which can lead to an incorrect diagnosis of Wilms' tumor. Such a situation occurs when there is hydronephrosis of the upper moiety, with no caliceal filling in the enlarged upper pole but with normal lower calices (Figure 7). Solitary cyst of the kidney, quite different in children from the more common adult variety, usually takes the form of an enormous hydrocalix with gross destruction of renal parenchyma,[15] and differentiation from Wilms' tumor is not difficult.

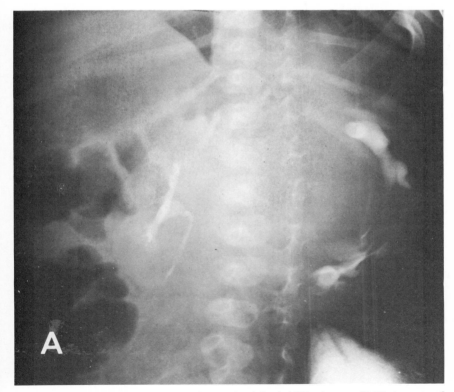

Figure 4. (A) Distortion of the pelvicaliceal system by a left-sided Wilms' tumor. (B) Displacement of an intact renal pelvis by a proven neuroblastoma. Note the bulge of the contralateral mediastinum due to metastases (arrow). (C) Invasion of the left renal pelvis by a proven intrarenal neuroblastoma.

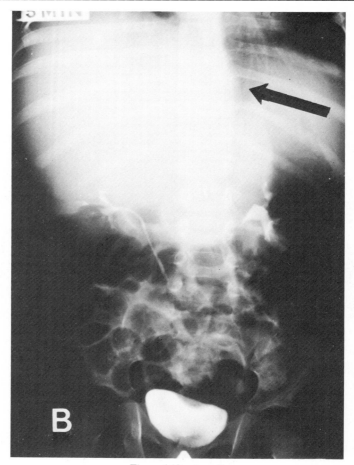

Figure 4 (Continued)

Medial displacement of the upper ureter around a lower pole tumor occurs in 15% of cases. Ureteral obstruction by the tumor is not seen. This sign may also be encountered in renal cell carcinoma.

Atypical features which are uncommon in Wilms' tumor are: (1) a nonfunctioning kidney, (2) defuse renal enlargement, (3) pelvic hydronephrosis, (4) obliteration of a calix, and (5) filling defects in the pelvis or calices.

Retrograde Pyelography

This procedure will usually not be indicated in Wilms' tumor since complete

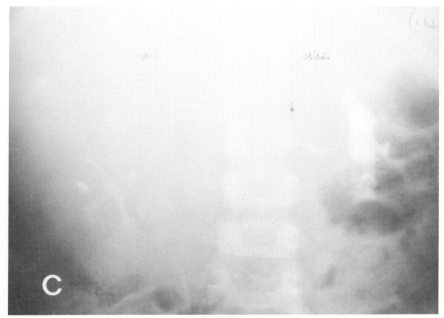

Figure 4 (Continued)

nonfunction is rare. Retrograde examination is not without risk and penetration of the tumor by the catheter can predispose to the dissemination of malignant cells.

Inferior Venacavography

This procedure may be combined with excretory urography with but little increase in the total time required for the examination. The procedure then becomes supplementary to pyelography, not competitive with it, and only a single film is added to the routine urogram. The child is mildly sedated, tourniquets are placed on both thighs just below the groins, and the long saphenous vein at the ankle is cannulated. Contrast medium, 10 to 20 ml, is injected manually as rapidly as possible and the tourniquet on the injected leg is removed when 75% of the injection is completed. A single film is taken from the pubis to the upper thorax, including the lower chest and the entire abdomen.

Deviation from the normal cavogram indicates a greater possibility of renal malignancy, and 90% of cases showing obstruction of the vena cava were malignant. The investigation also furnishes a useful guide to surgical respectability.[16] All cases of Wilms' tumor showed displacement of the inferior vena cava; smooth filling defects along the ipsilateral caval margin may also be seen. Unfortunately,

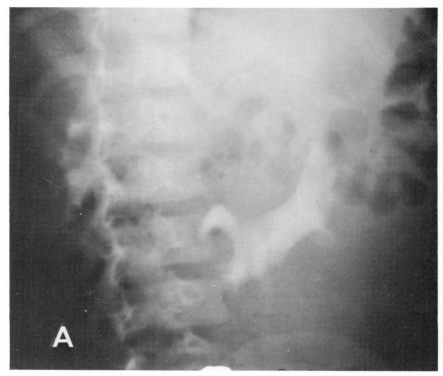

Figure 5. *(A)* Enlargement of the pelvicaliceal system and localized hydrocalycosis. *(B)* Enlargement of the pelvicaliceal system (arrow). *(C)* Dilatation of all the major calices.

there is a real incidence of false positives arising from a variety of artifacts; these include layering and streaming phenomena and divergence of contrast medium into normal collateral pathways.[17,18] Various techniques have been recommended to overcome these difficulties, including two separate injections[19] and bilateral, simultaneous injections with decubitus, delayed and biplane films.[20]

Arteriography

This procedure was rarely performed on children with abdominal tumors until recently, because such children are usually promptly explored surgically apter minimal investigation,[21] and because the procedure is technically more difficult in children.[22,23] However, the percutaneous transfemoral Seldinger technique is a practical procedure from the fourth day of life onward. Since large, avascular areas are common in Wilms' tumors, selective renal arteriograms are preferable.[9]

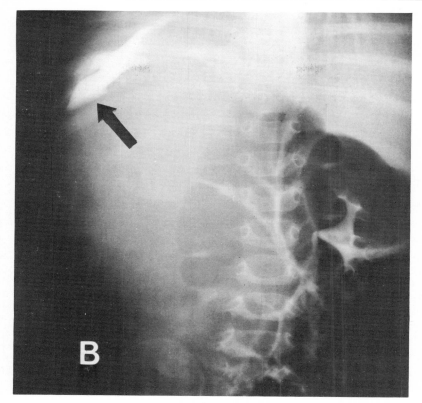

Figure 5 (Continued)

Arteriography is as informative for tumor evaluation in children as in adults[24] and has been more widely used for such purposes recently. This procedure is indicated when the diagnosis remains in doubt after urography and when immediate surgery is not the treatment of choice.[25]

Angiography (a) provides confirmatory evidence of a malignant tumor, (b) delineates the extent of the tumor and the involvement of adjacent structures, (c) defines the blood supply, reveals displacements of the renal pedicle and displays anomalous vessels, and (d) demonstrates tumor masses and metastases that were unsuspected.[9] Since 15% of patients with Wilms' tumor appear to have bilateral neoplasms,[26] the possible finding of a second and unsuspected tumor warrants serious consideration for the use of arteriography.[27]

Displacement of the aorta, with compression and stretching of the renal arteries by the neoplasm, appears to be invariable in Wilms' tumor. A florid tumor

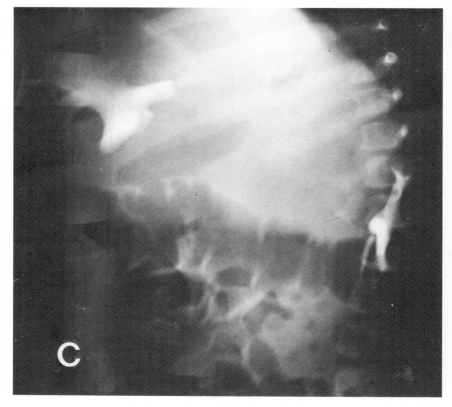

Figure 5 (Continued)

circulation (Figure 8), abnormal vessels of irregular caliber showing abrupt directional changes, arteriovenous anastomoses and pooling of contrast medium within the tumor mass in the venous phase are reported by most authorities.[8,9,28,29] A fine nodularity of tumor vessels may also be seen.[30]

In neuroblastoma, angiography confirms the urographic findings and usually demonstrates an extrarenal blood supply to the tumor, which invariably has a much more profuse vascularity than does Wilms' tumor. An absent or markedly hypoplastic renal artery, with no collateral arterial supply and no nephrogram, is a characteristic of the congenital multicystic kidney.[11] Highly typical vascular changes are seen in cases of renal dysplasia with thin, elongated and attenuated "spider-leg" and tortuous "corkscrew" vessels.[7] The defects in the nephrogram due to cysts that are common in hamartoma are clearly displayed by angiography. A pathognomonic vascular pattern, with characteristic "beaded" vessels, is seen less

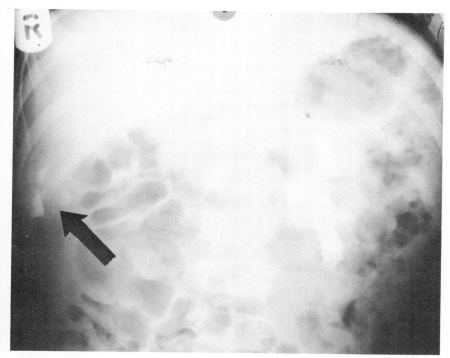

Figure 6. Late appearance of contrast medium in the form of rounded pools in the superolateral aspect of a right-sided Wilms' tumor (arrow).

frequently. Cysts or tumors may be shown in other areas such as liver and pancreas, by a midaortic injection.[31]

Transumbilical angiography may be useful in the investigation of the newborn infant with an abdominal mass. It is usually possible to catheterize the umbilical artery up to the fifth day after birth, and the technique has been described fully.[32] The occurrence of a single artery in the umbilical cord is associated with an increased incidence of other congenital abnormalities, including renal dysplasia.[33]

Phleboarteriourography has been claimed to represent a safe, simple, and quick method of examining children with abdominal tumors.[34] Contrast medium is injected into the femoral vein via a Teflon catheter and its course is followed through the venous, arterial, and urographic phases using a rapid film changer. In Wilms' tumor, the aorta and its principal branches are usually well opacified and the renal arteriogram is adequate. In cases with caval obstruction, however, in which the circulation is slowed and the arteriogram phase is useless because of contrast dilution, the nephrogram and urogram are excellent.

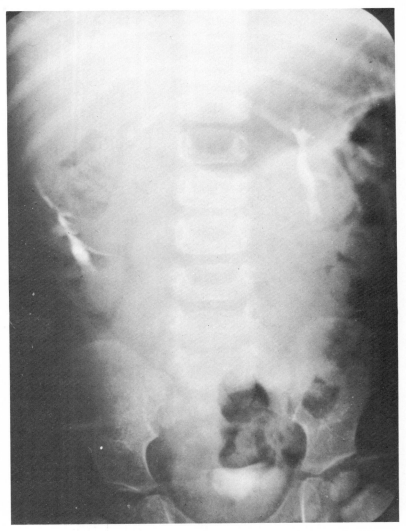

Figure 7. Normal lower calices but no caliceal filling in the enlarged right upper pole. This was a case of duplex kidney with gross hydronephrosis of the upper moiety.

ULTRASONOGRAPHY

This technique is very useful diagnostically in renal disease, especially when performed in close combination with excretory urography. It is indicated when renal nonfunction occurs at urography and in differentiating between cystic and

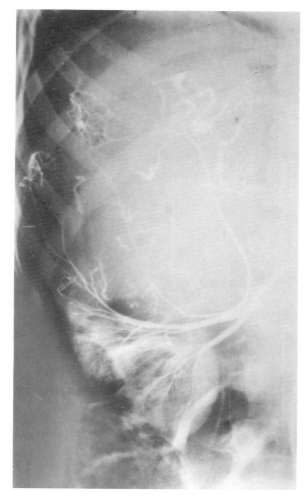

Figure 8.   Selective renal arteriogram showing a malignant circulation.

solid masses.[35] It should be employed as a preliminary to more complex investigations.[36]

The sonar diagnosis of Wilms' tumor has been fully reported.[37] The tumor appears in the A-scan as a large homogeneous area and in the B-scan as an extensive echo-free zone; in neither scan is it distinguishable from intact, normal renal parenchyma. However, additional scattered strong echoes within the tumor, probably caused by necrosis, are not uncommon. These echoes, together with acoustically different signals from weaker reflecting structures surrounding the tumor, may achieve a distinction between tumor and normal renal parenchyma. Good differentiation from echo-free fluid-containing masses, such as hydronephrosis and various cystic conditions, is readily achieved. It should be stressed that sonar can be easily employed even with seriously ill small children; there is a minimum of patient discomfort and no patient risk. Sonar is also useful after diagnosis in the assessment of tumor shrinkage with radiotherapy.

ISOTOPE SCANS AND RENOGRAPHY

It has been claimed that an isotope scan should routinely accompany excretory urography in the examination of the child with an upper abdominal mass.[38,39] There is no requirement for patient preparation and many of the technical difficulties encountered with urography are avoided. Isotope renography is said to be more sensitive and informative in the newborn and function not shown at urography may be demonstrated.[40,41] This may have considerable significance in the diagnosis of Wilms' tumor. The following findings have been reported in Wilms' tumor[39]: There is an irregular decrease in tubular uptake but total nonfunction is rare. Renal enlargement, with an irregular renal outline is common as is displacement of the kidney above or below an area of reduced isotope uptake.

The phenomenon of liver distortion of an extrinsic tumor can give rise to diagnostic difficulties. Wilms' tumor can be enormous, leading to considerable liver compression. Several cases have been reported in which Wilms' tumor patients were believed to have a hepatic tumor after liver scanning.[42]

Chest x-ray and bone scan should always be included in any diagnostic workup. Intrapulmonary metastases may be massive and are frequently present at diagnosis. Bony secondaries, however, unlike neuroblastoma, are relatively rare.

CONCLUSIONS

The vast majority of patients with Wilms' tumor are readily and correctly diagnosed. Hence, when a child presents with a clinical picture suggesting Wilms' tumor, immediate excretion urography is indicated; modified inferior vena cavography can easily be incorporated, and a chest film is essential. When the findings on the preliminary film and on the urogram are typical of Wilms' tumor, further radiography should be restricted to a search for metastases and urgent exploration, before or after chemotherapy and radiotherapy, is the ideal management.

In those cases in which the findings are atypical, the presence of a Wilms' tumor will be unlikely and further investigation is essential. This includes isotope studies and sonar examination, if immediately available, and retrograde pyelography if the kidney under suspicion is nonfunctioning. If the diagnosis is still in doubt, selective renal arteriography should be undertaken.

The diagnostic difficulties posed by the occurrence of Wilms' tumor in older age groups are entirely different. The tumor is rarely found in adolescents[43] or adults[44] and, when it does occur, it may present an atypical urographic appearance. Thus negative errors in diagnosis are likely, quite the reverse of the dangers of overdiagnosis in younger age groups. Full radiologic investigation is undertaken in practice to establish the diagnosis. Several cases have been reported following trauma,[45] and it is well known that diseased kidneys at all ages are prone to injury, often from minimal trauma.[46]

REFERENCES

1. Klapproth, H. J.: Wilms' tumour: A report of 45 cases and an analysis of 1351 cases reported in the World Literature from 1940 to 1958. *J. Urol.* 81:633–647, 1959.

2. Whiteside, C. G.: Radiological methods; pyelography and arteriography. In Riches, Sir E.: *Tumours of the Kidney and Ureter*, Livingstone, Edinburgh and London, 1964, p. 197.

3. Abeshouse, B. S.: Management of Wilms' tumour as determined by National Survey and Review of Literature. *J. Urol.* 77:792–813, 1957.

4. Lister, J., and Levick, R. K.: Errors in diagnosis in Wilms' tumour. *J. Pediatr. Surg.* 1:488–497, 1966.

5. Black, W. C., and Ragsdale, E. F.: Wilms' tumour. *Am. J. Roentgenol.* 103:53–60, 1968.

6. Hope, J. W., and Borns, P. F.: Radiologic diagnosis of primary and metastatic cancer in infants and children. *Radiol. Clin. North Am.* 3:353–374, 1965.

7. Cremin, B. J., and Kaschula, R. O.: Arteriography in Wilms' tumour; the results of 13 cases and comparison with renal dysplasia. *Br. J. Radiol.* 45:425–422, 1972.

8. Moes, C. A. F., and Burrington, J. D.: The use of aortography in the diagnosis of abdominal masses in children. *Radiology* 98:59–67, 1971.

9. McDonald, P., and Hiller, H. G.: Angiography in abdominal tumours in childhood with particular reference to neuroblastoma and Wilms' tumour. *Clin. Radiol.* 19:1–18, 1968.

10. Griscom, N. T.: Roentgenology of neonatal abdominal masses. *Am. J. Roentgenol.* 93:447–463, 1965.

11. Kyaw, M. M.: The radiological diagnosis of congenital multicystic kidney; "radiological triad." *Clin. Radiol.* 25:45–62, 1974.

12. Cope, J. R., Roylance, J., and Gordon, I. R. S.: The radiological features of Wilms' tumour. *Clin. Radiol.* 23:331–339, 1972.

13. Love, L., Neumann, H. A., Szanto, P. B., and Novak, G. M.: Malignant renal tumours in adolescence. *Radiology* 92:855–860, 1969.

14. Greenburg, L. A., McAlister, W. H., and Kissane, J.: Cystic disease of the kidneys in children. *Am. J. Roentgenol.* 100:135–146, 1967.

15. De Weerd, J. T., and Simon, H. B.: Solitary cyst of the kidney. *J. Urol.* 75:912–921, 1956.

16. Allen, J. E., Morse, T. S., Frye, T. R., and Clatworthy, H. W.: Vena cavograms in infants and children. *Ann. Surg.* 160:568–574, 1964.

17. Berdon, W. E., Baker, D. H., and Santulli, T. V.: Factors producing spurious obstruction of the inferior vena cava in infants and children with abdominal tumours. *Radiology* 88:111–116, 1967.

18. Doppman, J., Foley, H. T., and Hammond, W.: Inferior vena caval compression; the pseudo-obstruction syndrome. *Am. J. Roentgenol.* 100:411–416, 1967.

19. Tucker, A. S.: The roentgen diagnosis of abdominal masses in children; intravenous urography versus inferior vena cavography. *Am. J. Roentgenol.* 95:70–90, 1965.

20. Gabriele, O. F., Bell, O., and Martineau, R.: Pitfalls in inferior vena cavography. *Am. J. Roentgenol.* 100:417–423, 1967.

21. Hope, J. W., Borna, P. F., and Koop, C. E.: Diagnosis and treatment of neuroblastoma and embryoma of the kidney. *Radiol. Clin. North Am.* 1:543–621, 1963.

22. Sutton, D.: *Arteriography*, Livingstone, Edinburgh and London, 1962, pp. 34, 35, 160.

23. Haghighi, O., and Zimmerman, H. A.: Intravascular catheterisation, 2nd ed., Charles C Thomas, Springfield, 1966, p. 72.

24. Desilets, D. T., Ruttenberg, H. D., and Hoffman, R. B.: Percutaneous catheterisation in children. *Radiology* 87:119–122, 1966.

25. Chien-Hsing, M., and Elkin, M.: Angiographic manifestations of Wilms' tumour. *Am. J. Roentgenol.* 105:95–104, 1969.

26. Jagasia, K. H., Thurman, W. G., Pickett, E., and Grabstalot, H.: Bilateral Wilms' tumours in children. *J. Pediatr.* 65:371–376, 1964.

27. Silverman, F. N.: Paediatric radiology. In McLaren, J. W. (Ed.): *Modern Trends in Diagnostic Radiology*, 4th ser., Butterworths, London, 1970, p. 66.

28. Folin, J.: Angiography in Wilms' tumour. *Acta Radiol. Diagn.* 8:201–205, 1969.

29. Meng, C. H., and Elkin, M.: Angiographic manifestations of Wilms' tumour. *Am. J. Roentgenol.* 105:95–104, 1969.

30. Farah, J., and Lofstrom, J. E.: The angiography of Wilms' tumour. *Radiology* 90:775–777, 1968.

31. Wright, F. W., Ledingham, J. G. G., Dunnill, M. S., and Grieve, N. W. T.: Polycystic kidneys, renal hamartomas, their variants and complications. *Clin. Radiol.* 25:27–43, 1974.

32. Philip, T., Cockburn, F., and Anderson, J. M.: Abdominal aortography in the newborn via the umbilical artery. *Clin. Radiol.* 24:54–61, 1973.

33. Feingold, M., Fine, R. N., and Ingall, D.: Intravenous pyelography in infants with single umbilical artery. *N. Engl. J. Med.* 270:1178–1180, 1964.

34. Cecile, J. P., Fournier, A., Lelong, M., et al.: Phleboarterio-urography in the diagnosis of abdominal masses in children. *Clin. Radiol.* 23:340–348, 1972.

35. Holm, H. H.: Ultrasonic scanning in the diagnosis of space-occupying lesions of the upper abdomen. *Br. J. Radiol.* 44:24–36, 1971.

36. Damascell, B., Lattuada, A., Musumeci, R., and Severini, A.: Two-dimensional ultrasonic investigations of the urinary tract. *Br. J. Radiol.* 41:837–843, 1968.

37. Hünig, R., and Kinser, J.: Ultrasonic diagnosis of Wilms' tumors. *Am. J. Roentgenol.* 117:119–127, 1973.

38. Shuler, S. E., Meckstroth, G. R., and Maxfield, W. S.: The scintillation camera in paediatric renal disease. *Am. J. Dis. Child.* 120:115–121, 1970.

39. Samuels, L. D.: Scans in children with renal tumours. *J. Urol.* 107:127–132, 1972.

40. Kathel, B. L.: Radio-isotope renography as a renal function test in the newborn. *Arch. Dis. Child.* 46:314–320, 1971.

41. O'Neill, J. A., and Maxfield, W. S.: I-hippuran camera renogram for detection of urologic pathology in the newborn. *J. Pediatr. Surg.* 7:236–242, 1972.

42. Fellows, K. E., and Tefft, M.: Liver scans in children; abdominal masses simulating metastatic disease. *Am. J. Roentgenol.* **104**:678–681, 1968.

43. Lucke, B., and Schlumberger, H. G.: Tumours of the kidney, renal pelvis and ureter. In *Atlas of Tumour Pathology*, Sec. VIII, Fasc. 30, Armed Forces Institute of Pathology, Washington, D.C., 1957, pp. 10–17.

44. Snyder, W. H., Hastings I. N., and Pollock, W. F.: In Mustard, W. T., et al. (Eds.): *Pediatric Surgery*, (Vol. 2), *Retroperitoneal Tumours*. Year Book Medical Publishers, Chicago, 1969, pp. 1025–1028.

45. Fraley, E. E., and Halverstadt, D. B.: Unsuspected Wilms' tumour; danger in the conservative therapy of renal trauma. *N. Engl. J. Med.* **275**:373–374, 1966.

46. Slade, N., Evans, K. T., and Roylance, J.: The late results of closed renal injuries. *Br. J. Surg.* **49**:194–197, 1961.

CHAPTER FOUR

Immunologic Studies in Wilms' Tumors

PIERRE BURTIN, M.D., Ph.D.

Head of the Immunochemistry Laboratory and Associate Director
Institut de Recherches Scientifiques sur le Cancer
Villejuif, France

CONTENTS

A s with many other human tumors, one wonders whether nephroblastomas bear tumor-specific or tumor-associated antigens that are capable of inducing an antitumor immunity. Several authors studied these problems using various methods. Their results merit analysis, although they were sometimes incomplete or inconclusive. For the sake of clarity, we shall describe first the results of immunochemical experiments and then those of antitumor immunity studies.

IMMUNOCHEMICAL EXPERIMENTS

These experiments were based on the production of specific antisera in animals, generally rabbits, with nephroblastoma extracts, either individual or pooled. These extracts contained many normal components, either from the blood or the normal kidney structures present in the tumor. Thus it was necessary to carefully absorb the antisera with normal plasma, red cells, and normal kidney extracts. The antibodies that remained after such absorptions were studied by various methods such as immunodiffusion and immunofluorescence. A comparison was made between the reactivity of these antisera with tumor and with fetal extracts.

One might recall here that there is a succession of three embryonic and fetal kidneys during gestation. The last one, the metanephros, can be easily studied since it is present from the third month of gestation. The mesonephros, which is found during the second month of embryonic life is rarely available, and because of its small size it can only be studied by immunofluorescence. Work on the pronephros can be performed only on material obtained in the first month of gestation, which makes it virtually impossible to study. Thus the comparison between nephroblastoma and embryonic and fetal kidney extracts can never be complete.

In 1969, Linder[1] was the first to use immunochemical methods in this field. His study of 13 nephroblastomas led to results of varying importance. First, he characterized normal organ antigens in nephroblastoma, that are found either in other organs such as liver, spleen, thymus, lung and/or small intestine, or kidney specific. Some of these antigens were found in association with differentiated renal structures, that is, glomeruli or tubules, a few of them still present even in undifferentiated nephroblastoma. These latter antigens were localized by immunofluorescence in different morphologic areas. Thus antisera which stained the brush border of normal, proximal secreting tubules bound to cancerous tubular structures, and those reacting with normal glomerular epithelium stained the tumorous pseudoglomeruli.

A number of antigens present in normal kidney were absent in nephroblastomas. Thus, antiserum against normal kidney extracts absorbed with nephroblastoma extracts gave from five to eight precipitin lines with the immunizing extracts. (The number of lines given by the unabsorbed antiserum was not mentioned.)

These findings were confirmed by immunofluorescence studies which showed the absence of "kidney-specific" brush border antigens in nephroblastoma tubules when using an antikidney antiserum absorbed by small intestine extract.

Another finding of this study was the regular absence from the nephroblastoma of feto-specific antigens, such as α-fetoprotein. (The presence of carcinoembryonic antigen [CEA] was not investigated.) However, a fetal kidney antigen was found in 2 of the 13 nephroblastoma extracts. Finally, Linder was unable to characterize any tumor-specific antigen, since his antitumor antisera were completely absorbed by normal kidney extracts.

Since 1970, Allerton and his associates[2] have focused on an abnormal mucopolysaccharide found in the blood and urine of three children with Wilms' tumor. This component could be classified as an acid mucopolysaccharide, since it was precipitated by 3% acetic acid and was stained by Alcian blue. It also had a protein moiety. Its electrophoretic mobility was that of a prealbumin, and its sedimentation constant was estimated to be 2.7S. Its presence in large amounts in the blood of the three cancerous children was thought to be responsible for some biological abnormalities, such as high sedimentation rate, RBC rouleaux formation, and even prolonged clotting time. The tumors of the same patients, when extracted by EDTA or trypsin, contained a significant quantity of acid mucopolysaccharides biochemically similar to those of the blood. This suggested a tumoral origin of the blood component. Additional evidence favoring the intratumoral synthesis of this component was its rapid disappearance from the blood after tumor excision and its reappearance in the case of recurrence of tumor or metastasis. Allerton reviewed several reports[3,4] in the literature dealing with the presence of acid mucopolysaccharides, sometimes characterized as hyaluronidase sensitive, in the blood of patients afflicted with a nephroblastoma. Similar substances were also present in a neuroblastoma and a reticulum cell sarcoma.

Later, the same group undertook an immunochemical study of EDTA nephroblastoma extracts rich in acid mucopolysaccharides.[5] The antisera they had prepared gave two precipitin lines with the immunizing extracts, after absorption with whole blood and normal kidney extracts. One of these precipitin lines stained by Alcian blue was also given by the 3% acetic acid tumor precipitate. The authors did not report the frequency of these antigens in tumors, nor their presence in patients' sera. They described a cross-reaction between the antigen not precipitated by acetic acid and bovine fetuin.[6] In a recent paper (*Int. J. Cancer*, 1975, 16, 199–240, they showed the presence of this fetuin-like antigen in six rephroblastoma extracts.

The results in our laboratory,[7,8] are different from those mentioned above. First, we looked for acid mucopolysaccharides in a great number of nephroblastoma sera but rarely found them. We then concluded that searching for acid mucopolysaccharides in the blood is of little or no value for the diagnosis of Wilms' tumor.

Using immunochemical techniques we were able to find one tumor-specific antigen that we called "W" (for Wilms).[7] This antigen was demonstrated by an antiserum prepared with EDTA extracts of homogeneized nephroblastoma, and which was absorbed with normal human plasma, red cell stroma, and normal kidney extracts. Some of the EDTA extracts gave a strong precipitin line with the absorbed antiserum in Ouchterlony and immunoelectrophoretic plates; a very long line spreading over the whole β and α areas was then obtained (Figure 1). Other extracts were less rich in W-antigen. Thus it was necessary to use concentrated extracts prepared with phytic (inositol hexaphosphoric) acid and to employ a more sensitive technique, such as counter immunoelectrophoresis, to get a positive reaction. Even with more sensitive techniques, however, some nephroblastoma extracts did not contain detectable amounts of W-antigen.

We could not find W-antigen in normal kidney, either from the adult or the fetus. (Both the metanephros and the mesonephros were studied, the latter only by immunofluorescence.) Also, we could not find W-antigen in normal organs such as liver, spleen, lung, and so on. On the other hand, W-antigen was demonstrated by immunodiffusion techniques in some out of many carcinomas of other organs (e.g., breast, stomach) studied.

W-antigen is very resistant to proteolytic enzymes. Its precipitin line is stained by the periodic acid–Schiff reagent and Alcian blue. It is probably a polysaccharide or a glycoprotein. It is a weak antigen which usually does not elicit good antisera, and has not yet been isolated. By immunofluorescence, W-antigen was located in the cytoplasm of malignant cells and sometimes in extracellular deposits.

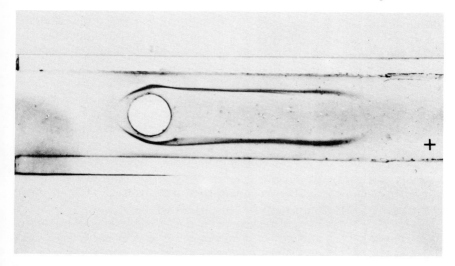

Figure 1. Immunoelectrophoretic analysis of a W-antigen, rich nephroblastoma extract reacting with anti-W antiserum.[7] The anode is on the right.

More recently, using immunochemical techniques, we identified another tumor-associated antigen in some nephroblastoma extracts. This new component does not react with anti-W antiserum, nor does its specific antiserum precipitate with W-antigen. No reaction was obtained between this latter antiserum and adult and fetal extracts either from kidney or other organs. This new antigen has some interesting features: it is a trypsin-sensitive glycoprotein of low molecular weight (about 20,000 to 30,000 daltons), and is notable for its very slow electrophoretic mobility (being found in the γ and post-γ areas). Since its strong antigenicity made it easy to obtain good antisera, we could prepare an immunosorbent according to the technique of Avrameas and Ternynck and use it to isolate small amounts of purified antigen suitable for radioactive labeling, in preparation for radioimmunoassay.

The significance of these two antigens is unknown. They do not react with the antisera specific for all the cancer-associated antigens studied so far: α-feto-protein, carcinoembryonic antigen of the digestive system, α 2H globulin, lactoferrin, or carcinofetal glial antigen. They are apparently not carcinofetal antigens, therefore their viral origin cannot be ruled out, and it is not unlikely that an unknown virus responsible for their synthesis could be the causative virus of the nephroblastoma. No comparison was made yet between our antigens and those described by Allerton's group.

ANTITUMOR IMMUNITY STUDIES

Two groups studied the action of lymphocytes that had been isolated from the peripheral blood of nephroblastoma-bearing patients and from control subjects on cultivated nephroblastoma cells. This action is generally called cytotoxicity, though it seems to be only cytostasis (inhibition of the multiplication) rather than true cell killing. The nephroblastoma cells were obtained by dissociation of surgically excised tumors which contained tumorous and nontumorous cells.

In 1971, Diehl et al.[9] were the first to study this problem. They obtained blood samples from 24 nephroblastoma-bearing patients and 24 age-matched controls. These included 7 healthy people, 9 noncancerous patients and 8 patients afflicted with a cancer other than nephroblastoma. The authors separated white blood cells by sedimentation, lysed red cells by 0.84% ammonium chloride, and purified mononuclear cells by filtration on a nylon wool column (or sometimes removed polymorphonuclear neutrophils by iron powder treatment). Pure lymphocytes were, however, obtained in only a few cases. Target cells originated from three nephroblastomas (two of them could be studied with the lymphocytes of their own patients) or from controls such as lung fibroblasts or normal kidney.

Thus various combinations have been tested in Takasugi and Klein microplates: nephroblastoma and control lymphocytes on nephroblastoma cells (of either the same or other patients) and on control cells. The ratio between lymphocytes and target cells varied from 2000:1 to 50:1.

Significant results were obtained. Control lymphocytes did not exhibit a specific cytotoxic effect, that is, they did not reduce the number of tumorous cells more than that of control cells. On the contrary, in almost half of the cases nephroblastoma lymphocytes were more cytotoxic on tumorous than on control cells, and the difference was significant. This effect was obtained with the lymphocytes of 8 out of 16 patients without metastasis, and in only 2 out of 8 patients with metastasis.

Kumar et al[10] made a parallel study of 11 nephroblastomas and 11 neuroblastomas in two series of criss-cross experiments. Their technique differed from that of Diehl et al. on several points. First, they separated the leukocytes from defibrinated blood by sedimentation in the presence of 3% gelatin, and sometimes they purified the lymphocytes by the method of Coulson and Chambers. They performed cytotoxicity experiments in small Petri dishes. The ratio of leukocytes to tumorous cells was as high as 5000:1 to 10,000:1. This could explain the high background; the number of Wilms' Tumor or neuroblastoma cells incubated with normal leukocytes was equally decreased by about 50%. On the other hand, nephroblastoma leukocytes reduced the number of autochtonous or allogeneic nephroblastoma cultivated cells by 79% and that of neuroblastoma cells by 50%. This difference was highly significant. Moreover, Kumar et al. found that leukocytes of two hypernephroma-bearing adult patients were also cytotoxic for nephroblastoma cells.

These two studies led to comparable results. They demonstrated a common, though not always present, reactivity between different nephroblastomas. These data are obviously similar to those obtained by the Hellströms, who were the first to show the organ specificity of in vitro antitumor cytotoxicity in human species. However, neither Diehl et al.[9] nor Kumar et al.[10] compared the cytotoxic action of nephroblastoma lymphocytes on nephroblastoma cells on one side and fetal kidney cells on the other side. Thus they did not reproduce the remarkable experiment in which the Hellströms[11] showed that the lymphocytes of colonic tumor patients were as cytotoxic on fetal intestine cells as on their own tumor cells. It is yet not known whether the antigen(s) common to many, if not all, nephroblastomas and able to sensitize patient's lymphocytes are also present in fetal kidney and are thus of the carcinoembryonic type.

These studies are interesting because they demonstrate an antitumor reactivity in nephroblastoma patients. At present, however, even strongly positive in vitro reactions do not allow one to infer an in vivo efficacy of the immune mechanisms. Thus it is necessary to be very cautious in generalizing from such results.

Surprisingly, there is no mention in the literature of studies of antitumor circulating antibodies. We examined the possible fixation of some nephroblastoma sera on nephroblastoma frozen sections by immunofluorescence, with negative results. Kumar (unpublished results), on the other hand, observed in a few nephroblastoma sera a factor capable of blocking lymphocyte cytotoxicity. This factor could be antitumor antibody, or free tumor antigen, or antigen-antibody complexes.

SUMMARY

Immunological studies on Wilms' tumor were often indicative of the existence of tumor-associated antigens and specific antitumor immunity. However, the results were never consistent. Furthermore, it is not yet clear whether both methods, immunochemistry and cytotoxicity, characterize the same antigens. This obviously indicates a direction for future research in this field.

ACKNOWLEDGMENTS

We are very grateful to Dr. Odile Schweisguth and Dr. Jean Lemerle, of the Children's Department of Institut Gustave Roussy, Villejuif, for their kind help and cooperation. Thanks to their efforts we were able to study more than 50 nephroblastomas.

REFERENCES

1. Linder, E.: The antigenic structure of nephroblastoma. *Int. J. Cancer* **4**:232–247, 1969.

2. Allerton, S., Beierle, J. W., Powars, D., and Basetta, L.: Abnormal extracellular components in Wilms' tumor. *Cancer Res.* **30**:679–683, 1970.

3. Deutsch, H. F.: Some properties of a human serum hyaluronic acid. *J. Biol. Chem.* **224**:767, 1957.

4. Morse, B. S., and Nussbaum, M.: The detection of hyaluronic acid in the serum and urine of a patient with nephroblastoma. *Am. J. Med.* **42**:996–1002, 1967.

5. Wise, K., Beierle, J., Allerton, S., and Powars, D.: Antigens from Wilms' tumor (abstr.). *Fed. Proc.* **30**:1279, 1974.

6. Beierle, J. W., Wise, K., Powars, D., et al.: Abnormal protein-polysaccharide complexes associated with Wilms' tumor. Abstract XIth International Cancer Congress, vol. 1, Florence, 1974, p. 349.

7. Burtin, P., and Gendron, M. C.: A tumor associated antigen in human nephroblastomas. *Proc. Nat. Acad. Sci (US)* **70**:2051–2054, 1973.

8. Burtin, P., and Gendron, M. C. In preparation, 1975.

9. Diehl, V., Jereb, B., Stjernsward, J., et al.: Cellular immunity to nephroblastoma. *Int. J. Cancer* **7**:277–284, 1971.

10. Kumar, S., Taylor, G., Steward, J. K., et al.: Cellular immunity in Wilms' tumor and neuroblastoma. *Int. J. Cancer* **10**:36–43, 1972.

11. Hellström, I., Hellström, K. E., and Shepard, T. H.: Cell mediated immunity against antigens common to human colonic carcinomas and fetal gut epithelium. *Int. J. Cancer* **6**:346–351, 1970

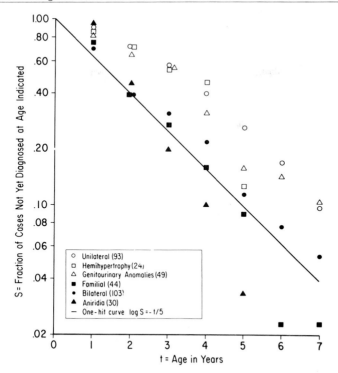

Figure 2. Semilogarithmic plots of fractions of cases of Wilms' tumor not yet diagnosed versus age in years. (Adapted from Knudson and Strong.[13])

familial Wilms' tumor among a total of 440 patients, many of whom did not have a complete family history. A frequency of familial cases of 1 to 2% is compatible with other recent surveys.[21-23, 25]

ASSOCIATION WITH CONGENITAL ANOMALIES

Development of a specific model to relate hereditary and nonhereditary Wilms' tumor offered an opportunity to analyze the association of Wilms' tumor with various congenital anomalies relative to genetic or teratogenic mechanisms. The association of Wilms' tumor with aniridia is much more frequent than expected, as aniridia was observed in 6 out of 440 patients with Wilms' tumor.[24] On the other hand, Wilms' tumor developed in one-third of patients with severe sporadic aniridia.[26] Analysis of 30 cases of Wilms' tumor associated with aniridia revealed that the Wilms' tumor occurred at an early age (Figure 2) and with a high frequency of bilaterality, a pattern similar to that of hereditary Wilms' tumor.[13] Recent reports have confirmed this pattern.[27-33]

These data suggest that the Wilms' tumor associated with aniridia is determined by a germinal mutation. Although aniridia itself may be determined by an autosomal dominant mutation,[34] aniridia in association with Wilms' tumor is generally sporadic and associated with severe congenital anomalies. It has been suggested[13] that the association of Wilms' tumor and aniridia might be the result of a new germinal mutation with pleiomorphic effects, or of mutation at the same locus operative in hereditary Wilms' tumor but including mutation of adjacent chromosomal loci. The latter phenomenon might be detectable grossly as a chromosomal abnormality.

Routine karyotyping on 7 patients with Wilms' tumor and aniridia[26,30,35] indicated no chromosomal abnormality. Recently, however, a case of Wilms' tumor and aniridia has been described[33] in which sophisticated, chromosomal banding techniques and computer analysis were required to demonstrate a chromosomal translocation t (8p+; llq−) with an interstitial deletion of the short arm of chromosome 8. This finding may be fortuitous and must be confirmed by additional reports. Nonetheless, the possibility that associated hereditary disorders may be due to deletion of adjacent loci is intriguing and invites comparison to the association of retinoblastoma and the D-deletion syndrome.[36,37] Present data suggest that identification of a specific chromosomal locus for a herditary tumor may be possible. It is interesting that each of the above-mentioned loci is on a different chromosome, ruling out any single chromosomal determinant for hereditary tumors.

Wilms' tumor is less frequently associated with another congenital anomaly, hemihypertrophy.[24] Analysis of 24 reported cases[13] (Figure 2) showed that when associated with hemihypertrophy, the age at diagnosis of Wilms' tumor did not differ from that of unselected cases, and in no case was the tumor bilateral. There was an excess of female patients with Wilms' tumor and hemihypertrophy[13,38,39] similar to that seen in hemihypertrophy in general.[40] Hemihypertrophy has also been associated with childhood tumors of the adrenal cortex and liver,[41] and with nonmalignant renal anomalies.[42-44] It may be that some endogenous or exogenous factors create an environment of stimulation and overgrowth that increases somatic mutation rates and thus increases the likelihood of malignancy. This phenomenon may explain the overlap among hamartomatous syndromes, hemihypertrophy, and childhood malignancy.[38,45]

Although hemihypertrophy is not associated primarily with the prezygotically determined Wilms' tumor, there is one family originally reported by Bishop and Hope[46] and recently reviewed by Meadows et al.,[20] in which 3 of 5 siblings had Wilms' tumor (bilateral in one, multifocal, unilateral in another), a fourth had a double urinary collecting system on one side, and the mother had asymmetry of the thumbs and feet. Although this could be a fortuitous occurrence, it might also indicate that the mother was a gene carrier for Wilms' tumor who manifested only hemihypertrophy. It is interesting to speculate that her Wilms' tumor may have spontaneously regressed. Association with the Wilms' tumor gene suggests that hemihypertrophy may be associated with some basic developmental abnormality characteristic of Wilms' tumor, irrespective of its pre- or postzygotic origin. In general, however, hemihypertrophy does not appear to represent a pleiomorphic effect of the Wilms' tumor gene, or an adjacent mutant locus. Hemihypertrophy appears to be associated with a higher than expected frequency of postzygotically determined tumor.

Wilms' tumor may also be associated with various genitourinary anomalies in the absence of any defined syndrome.[24] These anomalies are a heterogenous group including horseshoe kidney, anomalous urinary collecting systems, and genital anomalies such as pseudohermaphroditism, hypospadias, and cryptorchidism.[47-59] Analysis of the ages at diagnosis of 49 cases of Wilms' tumor in patients with genitourinary anomalies (Figure 2)[13] demonstrated that none of the above anomalies was consistently associated with the prezygotic form of Wilms' tumor.

Perhaps the association of Wilms' tumor with each genitourinary anomaly should be considered independently, as the etiology of the associations may differ. However, numbers of cases would then be too small to permit appropriate analysis. At this time it seems more likely that disordered events occurring during embryogenesis may lead or predispose both to specific genitourinary anomalies and Wilms' tumor. Any delay or inhibition of the maturation process in the renal blastema or related tissues may increase the possibility of somatic mutations and also permit persistence of the embryonal target tissue. Conversely, the presence of abnormal renal blastema or a precursor Wilms' tumor may predispose to abnormal embryologic development in related organ systems. The latter situation would lead to association of both pre- and postzygotic Wilms' tumor with genitourinary anomalies, an association which has been observed.[59]

There must be a number of embryologic influences on the development of Wilms' tumor that may lead to tumor expression or regression. Wilms' tumor is thought to originate from metanephric blastema which is normally induced at from 8 to 34 weeks of gestation and is no longer observed after 36 weeks gestation.[60] Consequently, any event or precursor state that may lead to the development of Wilms' tumor, hereditary or nonhereditary, must probably occur prior to the 36th week of gestation, and may be evident clinically.

There are certain diffuse disturbances in nephrogenesis that resemble Wilms' tumor histologically and have been noted as incidental autopsy findings in infants. These lesions have been referred to variously as "nephroblastoma in situ,"[61] "nephroblastomatosis,"[62] or "nodular renal blastema."[63] They have been found only in autopsy specimens of patients who died at less than 4 months of age, and in surgical or autopsy specimens of patients with Wilms' tumor.[63] Among those associated with Wilms' tumor, five of eight lesions occurred in patients with bilateral Wilms' tumor.[63] Similar lesions have been reported in specimens from patients with familial Wilms' tumor.[13] Thus, in older individuals the lesions seem to be associated with hereditary Wilms' tumor specimens. Further, in at least one family[64,65] this or a related condition occurred in 5 siblings of a consanguineous marriage of normal parents. However, the occurrence of these lesions in 0.25 to 0.5% of infants who died at less than 4 months[61,63] is difficult to reconcile with known mutation rates and the much lower frequency of clinical Wilms' tumor. This discrepancy suggests that either those infants represent an extremely high risk group for Wilms' tumor or that most such lesions spontaneously regress.

Indeed, there is reason to consider certain of the dying infants as members of an unusually high risk group because many have had trisomy 18[61,63,66] and "a unique condition of abnormal proliferation of cells assumed to derive from metanephric blastema accompanies the trisomy 18 syndrome."[63] At least one long-term survivor of trisomy 18 developed a Wilms' tumor.[67] Also there is an increased frequency of horeshoe kidneys and ureteral anomalies with trisomy 18, both with and without nodular renal blastema. This again suggests some common embryologic control mechanisms relating these genitourinary anomalies to disordered metanephric blastema. Certainly no conclusions as to the malignant potential of these lesions, or their specific relationship to pre- or postzygotic Wilms' tumor can be made. It would be of interest to know whether the incidence of nephroblastoma in situ is universally constant, as is the incidence of Wilms' tumor.

IMPLICATIONS FOR EPIDEMIOLOGIC STUDIES

Analysis of Wilms' tumor in general, in familial cases, and in association with various congenital anomalies has demonstrated that Wilms' tumor occurs in two distinct patterns of development. In one case the tumor develops early, is frequently multifocal, and is attributed to a prezygotic event. In the other case the tumor occurs later, is single, and is attributed to a postzygotic event. These two patterns should have relevance to epidemiologic studies and may be useful in identification of teratogenic agents. Given the present constancy of the development of Wilms' tumor, any change in its occurrence may serve as an index of changing environmental conditions. Any environmental variable might be evaluated by its effect, both on the overall incidence of Wilms' tumor and particularly on the incidence of pre- or postzygotically determined Wilms' tumor. A change in the proportion of each tumor type might be roughly measured by the change in the age at diagnosis of tumor or tumor multiplicity, but it is recognized that age at diagnosis may depend on cultural conditions and medical facilities. However, any change in germinal mutation rates in general, any change at the

Wilms' tumor locus in particular, or any change in the natural selection for Wilms' tumor gene carriers might be expected to produce an increased incidence of tumors of early onset and high frequency of multiplicity.

In the past the universally poor survival rate probably determined that this gene was maintained in the population primarily by new mutations occurring at a constant rate. The improved survival of patients with Wilms' tumor in medically advanced societies and their ability to reproduce may gradually affect a small change in the incidence of hereditary tumors. This has already been observed for retinoblastoma.[68] Likewise, any condition that changes prenatal somatic mutation rates in general, or disrupts embryogenesis in such a manner as to increase the probability of somatic mutation in the target tissue, might be expected to produce an increased incidence of single tumors of later onset.

One example of an agent known to increase somatic mutation rates per se is radiation. Intrauterine radiography is associated with an increased incidence of late onset (5 to 10 years of age) leukemia and solid tumors.[69,70] For retinoblastoma there is at least the suggestion that a specific agent may act on a specific tissue during embryogenesis to increase the likelihood of postzygotically determined malignancy. An area of increased incidence of unilateral, late onset retinoblastoma was identified and a relationship to endemic congenital trachoma infection[71] was proposed. Any area in which unilateral, late onset Wilms' tumor is noted to occur with a higher than expected incidence should be carefully examined for an etiologic association.

IMPLICATIONS FOR GENETIC COUNSELING

Many unknown factors affect tumor development and regression, gene fixation, penetrance, genetic regulation, mechanisms of gene action, and embryologic influences. Despite all these unknown factors, however, there are a number of clinical applications to management of patients with Wilms' tumor to be derived from the study of hereditary and nonhereditary Wilms' tumor. It should be recognized that in approximately 38% of cases, Wilms' tumor is initiated by a prezygotic event. The tumor then occurs as an autosomal dominant trait with a pentrance of approximately 63%, it occurs at an early average age, it is frequently multifocal, and it may occasionally be accompanied by severe sporadic aniridia. In the association of Wilms' tumor with severe sporadic aniridia a gross chromosomal deletion may have occurred. In the remaining 62% of cases, Wilms' tumor is initiated by a postzygotic event, occurs as a sporadic, invariably single tumor which develops at a later age, and may be associated with other congenital anomalies indicating postzygotic disordered embryogenesis.[13]

Recognition of the occurrence of prezygotic Wilms' tumor is important. Although the observed frequency of familial Wilms' tumor is only 1 to 2%, it has been estimated that 38% of cases are of prezygotic origin. The reason for this apparent discrepancy is that most hereditary cases are probably due to new mutations. In the absence of a family history of Wilms' tumor, or presenting multifocal Wilms' tumor, these patients are indistinguishable from Wilms' tumor patients in general except for an early average age at diagnosis. However, they have a unique, hereditary tumor predisposition and genetic counseling is definitely in order.

Each patient with the prezygotically determined Wilms' tumor is at risk for developing multiple primary foci of Wilms' tumor. Within his family, there is a minimum risk of 1 to 2% for siblings or first cousins to develop Wilms' tumor. Since the survival of Wilms' tumor has improved dramatically in the last 15 years,[72,73] genetic counseling concerning potential offspring is indicated for the increasing number of survivors. In the case of a patient with familial or bilateral Wilms' tumor, the risk of an affected offspring is simply computed by multiplying the 0.50 risk of transmitting an autosomal dominant gene times the 0.63 gene penetrance, which equals 0.32. For the more common case of a "sporadic," unilateral Wilms' tumor patient, the risk for an affected offspring can be estimated by multiplying the probability that the patient is a gene carrier, 0.38, times the risk of transmitting the mutant gene, 0.50, times the gene penetrance, 0.63, to yield a risk of 0.12. If the likelihood of an affected child being born to a survivor of Wilms' tumor is only 0.12, it is not surprising that no affected offspring were detected in a study of the progeny of childhood cancer survivors[74] among two offspring of two Wilms' tumor patients. However, further such studies are in order.

Twins present a special case for genetic counseling. For monozygous twins in general the expected concordance is 0.24, as determined by multiplying the probability that the tumor is of prezygotic origin, 0.38, times the gene penetrance, 0.63. Should one of monozygous twins develop a tumor of known prezygotic origin, as recognized by family history or bilaterality, the expected risk for the other twin would be the gene penetrance, 0.63.

There is a further risk with which survivors of Wilms' tumor must contend that may be of special importance to gene carriers: that is, their risk of developing other primary tumors. Irrespective of their genetic predisposition to tumor, most of these patients will be at some unknown but increased risk due to their exposure to carcinogenic x-ray therapy and potentially carcinogenic chemotherapy. However, again by analogy to retinoblastoma, there may be an increased susceptibility to certain specific tumors and/or to mutagenic agents among gene carriers.[75-77] There are many isolated reports of patients with Wilms' tumor who developed other primary tumors.[22,24,78-87] The only report from which any estimate of the frequency of other tumors might be made came from Mohr and Murphy,[22] who reported additional tumors in 3 out of 34 Wilms' tumor patients who survived over 5 years. However, until a systematic study of survivors can be carried out, it will be difficult to discern whether the number of additional tumors exceeds that expected by chance. Fortunately, international cooperation in registration and follow-up[5] should provide information more readily than that available from a single institution. Perhaps such cooperative studies will provide guidelines as to the hazards ahead for these survivors. Certainly a gene which predisposes to Wilms' tumor in early childhood may have pleiotropic effects not yet recognized.

The future for early cancer detection and prevention lies in identification of high-risk individuals prior to tumor development, and recognition of etiologic agents which contribute to tumor development. In the absence of detectable environmental variation in Wilms' tumor, one must concentrate on the identification of high-risk individuals. Those with a family history of Wilms' tumor, or with aniridia, hemihypertrophy or genitourinary anomalies, are at an increased risk for Wilms' tumor and should be appropriately counseled and followed. However, one must realize that even identification of all gene carriers prior to tumor development would recognize only 38% of patients in a pretumor state; the 62% of patients who develop tumor due to sequential postzygotic events would still be undetected until frank tumor appeared.

Thus it is most important to concentrate attention on identification and elimination of agents that may contribute to the postzygotic steps necessary for tumor development. However, spontaneous mutation of somatic cells will probably continue to maintain Wilms' tumor in the population at some baseline level of occurrence. If so, then one must accept Wilms' tumor as a persistent problem and continue to search for clues to early diagnosis and successful treatment.

SUMMARY

The development of Wilms' tumor has been attributed to two mutational steps, the first of which may occur in a germinal cell and result in hereditary Wilms' tumor, or in a somatic cell and result in nonhereditary Wilms' tumor. Hereditary Wilms' tumor is transmitted as an autosomal dominant disorder with 63% penetrance, occurs at an early average age, and may be bilateral. Nonhereditary Wilms' tumor occurs at a later age and is single. The hereditary form of Wilms' tumor is occasionally associated with severe aniridia, and may be related to a specific chromosomal deletion. The nonhereditary form of Wilms' tumor is occasionally associated with hemihypertrophy or genitourinary anomalies, suggesting some common control mechanisms during embryogenesis.

Recognition that not all Wilms' tumors are a homogeneous group in terms of etiology has important implications. Epidemiologic studies may be designed to identify factors influencing the development of a specific subgroup of Wilms' tumors. Genetic counseling may be instituted regarding the risk to the affected individual of other tumors, and the risk of Wilms' tumor in his siblings and offspring. The mutational model also has important implications for cancer control. Identification of gene carriers may lead to early tumor detection and/or prevention. Identification and elimination of agents that increase germinal or somatic mutation rates may lower the incidence of hereditary or nonhereditary tumors. However, spontaneous somatic mutation rates will always maintain a certain population of patients with Wilms' tumor which must be diagnosed and treated.

REFERENCES

1. Doll, R., Payne, P., and Waterhouse, J.: *Cancer Incidence in Five Continents*, Vol. 1, Springer-Verlag, Berlin, 1966.

2. Doll, R., Muir, C., and Waterhouse, J.: *Cancer Incidence in Five Continents*, Vol. II, Springer-Verlag, Berlin, 1970.

3. Editorial: Nephroblastoma: an index reference cancer. *Lancet* 2:651, 1973.

4. Innis, M. D.: Nephroblastoma: index cancer of childhood. *Med. J. Aust.* 2:322–323, 1973.

5. Miller, R. W.: Childhood cancer epidemiology: two international activities. *Natl. Cancer Inst. Monogr.* 40:71–74, 1974.

6. Davies, J. N. P.: Some variations in childhood cancers throughout the world. In Marsden, H., and Steward, J. (Eds.): *Tumours in Children*, Springer-Verlag, New York, 1968, pp. 13–36.

7. Fedrick, J., and Alberman, E. D.: Reported influenza in pregnancy and subsequent cancer in the child. *Br. Med. J.* 2:485–488, 1972.

8. Burkitt, D. P.: Etiology of Burkitt's lymphoma; an alternative hypothesis to a vectored virus. *J. Natl. Cancer Inst.* 42:19–28, 1969.

9. Herbst, A. L., Ulfelder, H., and Poskanzer, D. C.: Adenocarcinoma of the vagina: association of maternal stilbestrol therapy with tumor appearance in young women. *N. Engl. J. Med.* 284:878–881, 1971.

10. Miller, R. W.: Transplacental chemical carcinogenesis in man. *J. Natl. Cancer Inst.* 47:1169–1171, 1971.

11. Bourgoin, J. J., Cueff, J., Bailly, C., and Dargent, M.: Incidence de néphroblastomes chez le rat Sprague-Dawley immunodéprimé soumis au D.M.B.A. *Bull. Cancer* 59:429–434, 1972.

12. Ivankovic, S.: Intrauterine induction of cancer by the experimental application of chemical substances. *Recent Results Cancer Res.* 44:16–20, 1974.

13. Knudson, A. G., Jr., and Strong, L. C.: Mutation and cancer: a model for Wilms' tumor of the kidney. *J. Natl. Cancer Inst.* 48:313–324, 1972.

14. Knudson, A. G., Jr.: Mutation and cancer: statistical study of retinoblastoma. *Proc. Natl. Acad. Sci. US* 68:820–823, 1971.

15. Kaufman, R. L., Vietti, T. J., and Wabner, C. I.: Wilms' tumour in father and son. *Lancet* 1:43, 1973.

16. Brown, W. T., Puranik, S. R., Altman, D. H., and Hardin, H. C., Jr.: Wilms' tumor in three successive generations. *Surgery* 72:756–761, 1972.

17. Fitzgerald, W. L., and Hardin, H. C., Jr.: Bilateral Wilms' tumor in a Wilms' tumor family; case report. *J. Urol.* 73:468–474, 1955.

18. Leen, R. L. S., and Williams, I. G.: Bilateral Wilms' tumor; seven personal cases with observations. *Cancer* 28:802–806, 1971.

19. Kontras, S. B., and Newton, W. A., Jr.: Familial Wilms' tumor (Birth Defects–Original Articles Series). Fifth Conf. Nat. Found. March of Dimes 10:187–188, 1974.

20. Meadows, A. T., Lichtenfeld, J. L., and Koop, C. E.: Wilms' tumor in three children of a woman with congenital hemihypertrophy. N. Engl. J. Med. 291:23–24, 1974.

21. Aron, B. S.: Wilms' tumor; a clinical study of 81 patients. Cancer 33:637–646, 1974.

22. Mohr, R. R., and Murphy, G. P.: Wilms' tumor; 30-year review of cases in Buffalo. N.Y. State J. Med. 74:660–665, 1974.

23. Martin, J., and Rickham, P. P.: Wilms' tumour—an improved prognosis; report of 22 consecutive children seen from 1967–1971. Arch. Dis. Child. 49:459–462, 1974.

24. Miller, R. W., Fraumeni, J. F., Jr., and Manning, M. D.: Association of Wilms' tumor with aniridia, hemihypertrophy and other congenital malformations. N. Engl. J. Med. 270:922–927, 1964.

25. Ledlie, E. M., Mynors, L. S., Draper, G. J., and Gorbach, P. D.: Natural history and treatment of Wilms' tumour; an analysis of 335 cases occurring in England and Wales 1962–1966. Br. Med. J. 4:195–200, 1970.

26. Fraumeni, J. F., Jr., and Glass, A. G.: Wilms' tumor and congenital aniridia. JAMA 206:825–828, 1968.

27. Frauré, C., and Lange, J.-Cl.: Néphroblastome et aniridie. Ann. Radiol. 10:555–557, 1967.

28. Campinchi, R., Schweisguth, O., Blanck, C., and Lemerle, J.: Un nouveau cas d'association aniridie-néphroblastome. Bull. Soc. Ophthalmol. Fr. 70:885–887, 1970.

29. Ardouin, M., Ferrand, B., Le Marec. B., et al.: Aniridie; néphroblastome et malformations génitales. Bull. Soc. Ophthalmol. Fr. 71:809–813, 1971.

30. Le Marec, B., Lautridou, A., Urvoy, M., et al.: Un cas d'association de néphroblastome avec aniridie et malformations génitales. Arch. Fr. Pediatr. 28:457, 1971.

31. Haicken, B. N., and Miller, D. R.: Simultaneous occurrence of congenital aniridia, hamartoma, and Wilms' tumor. J. Pediatr. 78:497–502, 1971.

32. Neidhardt, M.: Wilms' tumor und aniridie—ein genetisch fixiertes syndrom? Klin. Paediatr. 184:312–317, 1972.

33. Ladda, R., Atkins, L., Littlefield, J., et al.: Computer-assisted analysis of chromosomal abnormalities: detection of a deletion in aniridia/Wilms' tumor syndrome. Science 185:784–787, 1974.

34. Shaw, M. W., Falls, H. F., and Neel, J. V.: Congenital aniridia. Am. J. Hum. Genet. 12:389–415, 1960.

35. Flanagan, J. C., and DiGeorge, A. M.: Sporadic aniridia and Wilms' tumor. Am. J. Ophthalmol. 67:558–561, 1969.

36. Orye, E., Delbeke, M. J., and Vandenabeele, B.: Retinoblastoma and long arm deletion of chromosome 13; attempts to define the deleted segment. Clin. Genet. 5:457–464, 1974.

37. O'Grady, R. B., Rothstein, T. B., and Romano, P. E.: D-group deletion syndromes and retinoblastoma. Am. J. Ophthalmol. 77:40–45, 1974.

38. Fraumeni, J. F., Jr., Geiser, C. F., and Manning, M. D.: Wilms' tumor and congenital hemihypertrophy; report of five new cases and review of literature. Pediatrics 40:886–899, 1967.

39. Balci, S., and Say, B.: Wilms' tumor and congenital malformations. Turk. J. Pediatr. 11:146–155, 1969.

40. Ringrose, R. E., Jabbour, J. T., and Keele, D. K.: Hemihypertrophy. Pediatrics 36:434–448, 1965.

41. Fraumeni, J. F., Jr., and Miller, R. W.: Adrenocortical neoplasms with hemihypertrophy, brain tumors, and other disorders. J. Pediatr. 70:129–138, 1967.

42. Roggensack, G., and McAlister, W. H.: Bilateral nephromegaly in a child with hemihypertrophy. *Am. J. Roentgenol.* 110:546–549, 1970.

43. Sprayregen, S., Strasberg, Z., and Naidich, T. P.: Medullary sponge kidney and congenital total hemihypertrophy. *N.Y. State J. Med.* 73:2768–2772, 1973.

44. Mankad, V. N., Gray, G. F., Jr., and Miller, D. R.: Bilateral nephroblastomatosis and Klippel-Trenaunay syndrome. *Cancer* 33:1462–1467, 1974.

45. Reddy, J. K., Schimke, R. N., Chang, C. H. J., et al.: Beckwith-Wiedemann syndrome; Wilms' tumor, cardiac hamartoma, persistent visceromegaly, and glomeruloneogenesis in a 2-year-old boy. *Arch. Pathol.* 94:523–532, 1972.

46. Bishop, H. C., and Hope, J. W.: Bilateral Wilms' tumors. *J. Pediatr. Surg.* 1:476–487, 1966.

47. Eliason, E. O., and Stevens, L. W.: Wilms' tumor in a horseshoe kidney. *Ann. Surg.* 119:788–790, 1944.

48. Firstater, M.: Embrioma en un riñon en herradura, en una niña de 15 meses; heminefrectonia transperitoneal. *Rev. Argent. Urol.* 24:365–370, 1955.

49. Lawlor, J. B., Lattimer, J. K., and Wolff, J. A.: Wilms' tumor in a horseshoe kidney. *Pediatrics* 23:354–358, 1959.

50. Beck, W. C., and Hlivko, A. E.: Wilms' tumor in the isthmus of a horsehoe kidney. *Arch. Surg.* 81:803–806, 1960.

51. Lathem, J. E., and Smith, K. H.: Wilms' tumor in a horseshoe kidney; a surviving case. *J. Urol.* 88:25–28, 1962.

52. Jagasia, K. H., Thurman, W. G., Pickett, E., and Grabstaldt, H.: Bilateral Wilms' tumors in children. *J. Pediatr.* 65:371–376, 1964.

53. Montagnini, R., Mancia, A., Crisci, E., and Emanuelli, M.: Tumore di Wilms su rene a ferro di cavallo. *Policlinico* 76:305–313, 1969.

54. Currie, D. P., Daly, J. T., Grimes, J. H., and Anderson, E. E.: Wilms' tumor; a clinical pathological correlation. *J. Urol.* 109:495–500, 1973.

55. Denys, P., Malvaux, P., Van den Berghe, H., et al.: Association d'un syndrome anatomopathologique de pseudohermaphrodisme masculin, d'une tumeur de Wilms, d'une nephropathie parenchymateuse et d'un mosaicisme XX/XY. *Arch. Fr. Pediatr.* 24:729–739, 1967.

56. Drash, A., Sherman, F., Hartmann, W. H., and Blizzard, R. M.: A syndrome of pseudohermaphroditism, Wilms' tumor, hypertension, and degenerative renal disease. *J. Pediatr.* 76:585–593, 1970.

57. Spear, G. S., Hyde, T. P., Gruppo, R. A., and Slusser, R.: Pseudohermaphroditism, glomerulonephritis with the nephrotic syndrome, and Wilms' tumor in infancy. *J. Pediatr.* 79:677–681, 1971.

58. Barakat, A. Y., Papadopoulou, Z. L., Chandra, R. S., et al.: Pseudohermaphroditism, nephron disorder and Wilms' tumor; a unifying concept. *Pediatrics* 54:366–369, 1974.

59. Jereb, B.: Bilateral nephroblastoma; a clinical review of 19 cases. *Acta Radiol. (Ther.)* 10:417–426, 1971.

60. Potter, E. L.: Development of the human glomerulus. *Arch. Pathol.* 80:241–255, 1965.

61. Shanklin, D. R., and Sotelo-Avila, C.: In situ tumors in fetuses, newborns and young infants. *Biol. Neonate.* 14:286–316, 1969.

62. Hou, L. T., and Holman, R. L.: Bilateral nephroblastomatosis in a premature infant. J. Pathol. *Bacteriol.* 82:249–255, 1961.

63. Bove, K. E., Koffler, H., and McAdams, A. J.: Nodular renal blastema; definition and possible significance. *Cancer* 24:323–332, 1969.

64. Liban, E., and Kozenitzky, I. L.: Metanephric hamartomas and nephroblastomatosis in siblings. *Cancer* 25:885–888, 1970.

65. Perlman, M., Goldberg, G. M., Bar-Ziv, J., and Danovitch, G.: Renal hamartomas and nephroblastomatosis with fetal gigantism; a familial syndrome. *J. Pediatr.* **83**:414–418, 1973.

66. Milligan, G. F., and Young, D. G.: Nephroblastoma in childhood. *Scott. Med. J.* **16**:317–321, 1971.

67. Geiser, C. F., and Schindler, A. M.: Long survival in a male with 18-trisomy syndrome and Wilms' tumor. *Pediatrics* **44**:111–115, 1969.

68. Editorial: The changing pattern of retinoblastoma. *Lancet* **2**:1016–1017, 1971.

69. Stewart, A. M., and Kneale, G. W.: Age-distribution of cancers caused by obstetric x-rays and their relevance to cancer latent periods. *Lancet* **2**:4–8, 1970.

70. Stewart, A.: The carcinogenic effects of low level radiation; a re-appraisal of epidemiologists methods and observations. *Health Phys.* **24**:223–240, 1973.

71. Fourtuny, I. E.: Unilateral retinoblastoma. *Lancet* **1**:422, 1973.

72. Sutow, W. W., Gehan, E. A., Heyn, R. M., et al.: Comparison of survival curves, 1956 versus 1962, in children with Wilms' tumor and neuroblastoma; report of the subcommittee on childhood solid tumors, solid tumor task force, National Cancer Institute. *Pediatrics* **45**:800–811, 1970.

73. Fraumeni, J. F., Jr., Everson, R. B., and Dalager, N. A.: Declining mortality from Wilms' tumour in the United States. *Lancet* **2**:48, 1972.

74. Li, F. P., and Jaffe, N.: Progeny of childhood-cancer survivors. *Lancet* **2**:707–709, 1974.

75. Jensen, R. D., and Miller, R. W.: Retinoblastoma: epidemiologic characteristics. *N. Engl. J. Med.* **285**:307–311, 1971.

76. Strong, L. C., and Knudson, A. G., Jr.: Second cancers in retinoblastoma. *Lancet* **2**:1086, 1973.

77. Kitchin, F. D., and Ellsworth, R. M.: Pleiotropic effects of the gene for retinoblastoma. *J. Med. Genet.* **11**:244–246, 1974.

78. Riedel, H. A.: Adrenogenital syndrome in a male child due to adrenocortical tumor; report of case with hemihypertrophy and subsequent development of embryoma (Wilms' tumor). *Pediatrics* **10**:19–27, 1952.

79. Glenn, J. F., and Rhame, R. C.: Wilms' tumor; Epidemiologic experience. *J. Urol.* **85**:911–918, 1961.

80. Cohen, J., and D'Angio, G. J.: Unusual bone tumors after roentgen therapy of children. *Am. J. Roentgenol.* **86**:502–512, 1961.

81. Tefft, M., Vawter, G. F., and Mitus, A.: Second primary neoplasms in children. *Am. J. Roentgenol.* **103**:800–822, 1968.

82. Regelson, W., Bross, I. D. J., Hananian, J., and Nigogosyan, G.: Incidence of second primary tumors in children with cancer and leukemia. *Cancer* **18**:58–72, 1965.

83. DiGeorge, A. M., and Harley, R. D.: The association of aniridia, Wilms' tumor, and genital abnormalities. *Arch. Ophthalmol.* **75**:796–798, 1966.

84. Salmon, M., Coignet, J., Raybaud, C., et al.: Succession d'un néphroblastome et d'un symphathoblastome chez un nourrisson. *Pediatrie* **25**:337–342, 1970.

85. Jereb, B., and Eklund, G.: Factors influencing the cure rate in nephroblastoma; a review of 335 cases. *Acta Radiol.* **12**:84–106, 1973.

86. Chabalko, J. J., Creagan, E. T., and Fraumeni, J. F., Jr.: Epidemiology of selected sarcomas in children. *J. Natl. Cancer Inst.* **53**:675–679, 1974.

87. Valdes-Dapena, M. A., Huff, D. S., and DiGeorge, A. M.: The association of congenital malformations and malignant tumors in infants and children. *Ann. Clin. Lab. Sci.* **4**:363–371, 1974.

CHAPTER SIX

Wilms' Tumor in Domesticated and Experimental Animals and *in vitro*

E. C. PIRTLE, M.D., Ph.D.

Microbiologist, Virological Research Laboratory
National Animal Disease Center
North Central Region, Agricultural Research Service
United States Department of Agriculture
Ames, Iowa

CONTENTS

A renal tumor of embryonal origin (nephroblastoma) has been reported in man and in many of the lower animals. In man, this tumor, known as Wilms' tumor,[1] is a rapidly growing, early metastasizing, highly aggressive embryonal neoplasm of very young children. The embryonal origin of Wilms' tumor was pointed up by the finding of bilateral nephroblastoma in a premature child who lived for 13 hours.[2] Because of histologic similarity, nephroblastomas of lower animals have often been called Wilms' tumor.[3] Throughout this chapter, however, the designation of Wilms' tumor is applied only to nephroblastomas in humans.

Regardless of the species in which nephroblastomas occur, there is general agreement that all elements of the tumor arise from primitive nephrogenic blastema[4] of mesodermal origin.[5] Even though nephroblastomas may present wide histological variations, all such tumors contain immature and abortive tubules and glomeruli contained in a connective tissue stroma.[6] It is the purpose of this chapter to consider: (1) spontaneous nephroblastomas in lower animals, (2) induction of nephroblastomas in lower animals experimentally, and (3) results obtained in *in vitro* investigations with Wilms' tumor and nephroblastomas of lower animals.

SPONTANEOUS NEPHROBLASTOMAS IN DOMESTICATED AND OTHER LOWER ANIMALS

Swine

Feldman[7] reported that nephroblastoma is the most common tumor in swine, and identified 46 nephroblastomas out of 86 swine tumors in his collection. Of Feldman's 46 cases, 43 of the tumors were directly associated with the kidney, and 3 were extranephric. One example of a swine nephroblastoma identified in this laboratory was both kidney-associated and extranephric (Figure 1). Photomicrographs of histologic sections of both areas are shown in Figures 2A and 2B. In another series of 941 swine tumors, Sullivan and Anderson[8] found about one-fourth were nephroblastomas, whereas one-half were malignant lymphomas. These authors found only nine instances in which the nephroblastomas had metastasized.

In a more recent survey, of 4,718,600 swine slaughtered in federally inspected abattoirs in the United States during a 1-month period in 1966, 205 cases of nephroblastoma were confirmed histopathologically. It was concluded from this survey that nephroblastoma is the most common tumor in swine. A solitary tumor was found in approximately 80% of cases and bilateral involvement was found in about 18% of cases.[9] As part of a tumor survey in farm animals in England during a 10-year period, Cotchin[10] identified 6 nephroblastomas out of 27 swine tumors

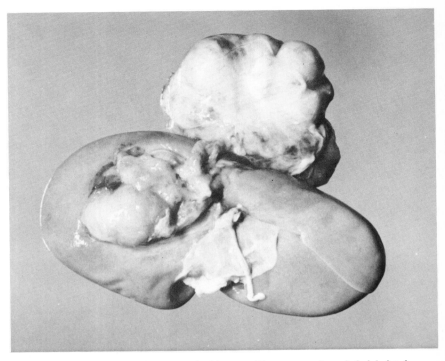

Figure 1. Gross specimen of a swine nephroblastoma. There are two irregularly lobulated masses associated with the kidney. One mass, 4 cm in diameter, is embedded in and rises above the anterior half of the kidney. The other mass, 6.7 cm in diameter, is attached superficially to the cortex along the greater curvature of the kidney and is largely extrarenal. The masses are connected by a band of tissue 0.5 cm wide, which appears to be part of the tumor.

examined, 2 from sows and 4 from 6- to 7-month-old young swine; lymphosarcoma was the most common tumor. The incidence and histopathology of primary renal tumors of swine encountered in a 1-year period in Great Britain revealed that 13 out of 16 tumors were nephroblastomas and 10 were from 5- to 9-month-old swine.[11] A nephroblastoma weighing 5 kg has been reported.[12]

Chickens

According to Feldman and Olson,[13] nephroblastoma is one of the more frequently occurring neoplasms in chickens. As with swine, most nephroblastomas in this species are unilateral and usually involve the kidney. In an earlier report,[14] the same authors reported a case of bilateral keratinized nephroblastoma without metastasis in a crossbred cockerel 10 months of age. Two cases of nephroblastoma which had not metastasized, but which had numerous mitotic figures were

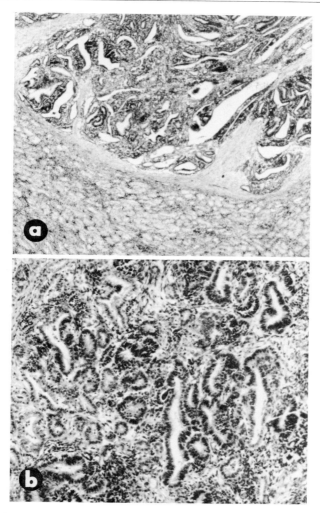

Figure 2. Photomicrographs of histologic sections of the kidney and extranephric areas of the nephroblastoma shown in Figure 1. (H/E stain). *(A)* Kidney showing an area of the nephroblastoma impinging on an area of normal kidney. A layer of fibrous connective tissue separates the tumor from the normal kidney (×40). *(B)* Extranephric area of the tumor showing numerous pseudotubular structures and nests of undifferentiated epithelium (×100).

reported by McKenney[15] in 1-year-old white leghorn hens. In their consideration of the avian leukosis complex, Helmboldt and Fredrickson[16] stated that avian nephroblastomas are of viral origin, may be transplanted, and never metastasize. However, Mathews[17] observed 12 cases of this tumor in chickens, and in 1 case there was metastasis to the left thigh, to the left lung, and to the right kidney. In addition to connective tissue, abortive tubules, and glomeruli, nephroblastomas may include areas of bone and cartilage.[18]

Cattle

As indicated in their examination of 302 renal tumors from cattle, Sandison and Anderson[11] found only 11 primary renal tumors, and only 1 was a nephroblastoma. As rare as this tumor appears to be in cattle, there are other reported cases, two of which point up the embryonal origin of spontaneous nephroblastomas. Walker[19] encountered a case of extranephric nephroblastoma in a 3-week-old calf in which there was no evidence of muscle, bone, or cartilage in histologic sections. Misdorp[20] recorded two cases of nephroblastoma in 6- to 7-month-old aborted bovine fetuses. One fetus had numerous abdominal tumors, and the other was kidney-associated. A similar report[21] was made in which a 6-month-old bovine fetus had a histologically confirmed case of nephroblastoma.

Rats

As various breeds of rats are used in laboratory investigations, spontaneous nephroblastomas in this species are of great importance to investigators. Bullock and Curtis[22] reported spontaneous embryonal carcinomas in their rat colony, the histologic descriptions of which are similar and compatible with those of nephroblastoma. Nephroblastoma without metastasis was detected in a 5-month-old Sprague-Dawley rat which was one of the principals in a preclinical toxicological study.[23] In a literature survey these same authors found that out of 49,869 necropsies performed on rats 2453 tumors were found, 23 of 31 renal tumors being nephroblastomas.

A case of metastasizing nephroblastoma in a 6-month-old Sprague-Dawley rat was reported from Sweden.[24] The point was made the tumor contained no striated muscle, cartilage, or bone. A spontaneous nephroblastoma in a 230-day-old albino rat was reported from Germany.[25] Pittermann[26] reported the occurrence of nephroblastoma encountered in each of 2 Sprague-Dawley and 2 Wistar specific pathogen-free rats; 3 were females. Aberrant glomerular and tubular formations were found when the tumors were examined histologically.

Dogs

The occurrence of nephroblastoma in dogs of various ages has been recorded. A neoplasm removed from a 5-year-old dachshund was identified histologically as a nephroblastoma.[27] As possibly the first case reported in a dog, the diagnosis was confirmed by three different pathologists. One interesting case in a 12-year-old Labrador bitch was reported.[28] In this instance the tumor as well as the involved omentum was removed surgically. However, due to metastasis to the mesentery, peritoneum, lung, hepatic and mediastinal lymph nodes, and thymus, the dog died. Histologic examination revealed numerous mitoses, and there was osteoid formation at the periphery of the pulmonary lesions, but not elsewhere. An exploratory laparotomy on an 8-month-old beagle bitch revealed a mass near the hilum of the right kidney. The kidney and tumor (a nephroblastoma) were removed.[29] Six weeks following surgery the beagle had radiologic evidence of metastasis to the lung. Nephroblastoma with metastasis to several sites was reported in a 9-year-old basenji dog.[30] A report from Germany of nephroblastoma in a 10-year-old German shepherd stressed that, despite the age of the dog, the tumor had not metastasized.[31]

Rabbits

Bell and Henrici[32] reported nephroblastomas in 2 rabbits (breed not mentioned) in which metastasis had not occurred and in which mitotic cells were not observed. Attempts to transplant the tumor to other rabbits via subcutaneous and intravenous routes, or to the kidney and anterior chamber of the eye were unsuccessful. Scott[33] recorded a case of nephroblastoma in a Belgian hare. The tumor had psuedotubular and glomerular structures, but no mitoses or metastases were observed. Greene[34] recorded the occurrence of rabbit nephroblastoma and was able to transplant the original tumor to the anterior chamber of the eye and to the testis of other rabbits. Tumor growth was more rapid in testicular tissue. Mitotic figures were common in involved eye and testicular tissues, but metastasis did not occur. Greene concluded that the rabbit tumors were not analogous to Wilms' tumor in humans.

Spontaneous nephroblastomas also have been reported in the cat,[35] goat,[36] sheep,[37] parakeet,[38] fire-bellied newt,[39] and striped bass.[40]

EXPERIMENTAL INDUCTION OF NEPHROBLASTOMAS IN LOWER ANIMALS

Transplantation

Rats. Toolan[41] reported successful heterotransplantation of human tumors in X-radiated and X-irradiated, cortisone-treated rats and hamsters. She succeeded in transplanting 90% of 101 human tumors to X-irradiated cortisone-treated rats; approximately the same results were obtained in rats receiving only cortisone. Successful heterotransplantation of a Wilms' tumor was achieved in X-irradiated, X-irradiated, cortisone-treated, and cortisone-treated rats. The tumor did not survive in untreated rats. It was subsequently reported[42] that human neoplasms could be maintained in series in cortisone-treated rats and hamsters. In addition, such routinely transplantable tumors also propagated well in cell culture and on the chorioallantoic membrane of embryonating chicken eggs.

A nephroblastoma arose spontaneously abutting the remaining kidney in a Sherman-Mendal rat that had undergone left nephrectomy at 2 months.[43] Histologically mitoses, tubular structures, and primitive glomeruli were present. A cell suspension of this tumor induced numerous sarcomatous nodules in a littermate rat after intraperitoneal inoculation. Another littermate developed sarcomatous peritoneal tumors after inoculation with a cell suspension from the first transplanted tumor. However, rats unrelated to the littermates failed to develop tumors after similar inoculations.

A female Wistar breeder rat was thought to be pregnant, but when she did not deliver autopsy disclosed the presence of a large nephroblastoma which surrounded and distorted the left kidney.[44] No metastases were found and no other abdominal organs were invaded. The original tumor was transplanted in series by intraperitoneal inoculation into suckling rats. Metastasis was not observed in initial passages but occurred frequently at higher passage levels. A nephroblastoma of an inbred Furth/Wistar rat was passaged through twenty-five generations of similar rats.[45] As the transplantable tumor preferentially metastasized to the lung, it was suggested that this rat tumor offered a model system for the controlled study of a neoplasm that closely resembled Wilms' tumor in histologic appearance and secondary metastatic lesions.

Hamsters. Syrian golden hamsters *(Mesocricetus auratus)* have been widely used as laboratory animals since they were first found in the wild, and after it was learned that they breed well in captivity.[46,47] The value and advantages of the cheek pouch of the Syrian hamster as the site for transplanting tumors were determined more than 20 years ago[48,49]: a high percentage of "takes" is achieved, tumors grow freely without physical hindrance, tumors can be observed frequently as growth progresses, and microscopic study of early stages of growth and vascularization can be made employing transillumination. Even though no reference was found for the occurrence of spontaneous nephroblastomas in hamsters, the Syrian hamster has been a valuable host for the propagation of a variety of human tumors,[50-54] including Wilms' tumors[55,56] and cell cultures derived from Wilms' tumors.[57,58]

The Syrian hamster appears somewhat unique in its ability to differentiate malignant from nonmalignant tissue. This ability was well exemplified by Foley and Handler[59] who studied the reactions in cortisone-treated and untreated hamsters of tissue culture cell lines derived from malignant and nonmalignant tissue. All cell lines grew in cortisone-treated hamsters if 1,000,000 or more cells were implanted in the cheek pouch. Cell lines derived from malignant tissues induced tumors when about 10 cells were inoculated, while those from normal tissue did not survive and grow if the inoculum had fewer than 1000 cells. This difference was even more striking when normal untreated hamsters were used. Cell lines derived from malignant tissues induced tumors after inoculation of 1000 or fewer cells, but cell lines from adult nonmalignant tissues failed to grow if fewer than 100,000 or 1,000,000 cells were inoculated. Normal embryonal tissue culture cell lines appeared to be intermediate between malignant and nonmalignant cell cultures in ability to survive and induce tumors. The authors suggest that these differences in growth potential represent inherent differences in capacity for autonomous growth in this heterologous host.[59]

Mice. An experimentally produced nephroblastoma in inbred strain 129/SV mice was reported[60] which resembled Wilms' tumor developmentally and histologically and which metastasized to the periaortic lymph nodes and lung. The tumors were induced by transplanting fetal renal blastemas of 129/SV mice to testes of adult mice of the same strain, that is, isogeneic transplantation. Viruses could not be identified either in cell cultures, or by electron microscopy of renal blastema, or in ensuing induced tumors. The authors concluded that the production of nephroblastoma with renal blastema supports the hypothesis that Wilms' tumor originates from metanephric blastema.

Viruses

As was mentioned earlier, spontaneous nephroblastomas occur in chickens. However, evidence presented indicated that nephroblastomas may be induced in chickens experimentally following exposure to avian tumor viruses. Nephroblastomas arising from exposure to the BAI strain A myeloblastosis virus were observed after inoculation of tumor cell suspensions into pectoral muscles, or following intravenous inoculation of cell-free filtrates of virus-induced tumors.[61] The observed nephroblastomas occurred in addition to myeloblastosis, visceral lymphomatosis, and osteopetrosis in some chickens. After nine serial passages of cell suspension, the tumor apparently lost its ability to induce myeloblastosis. Likewise, cell-free filtrate from twelfth passage tumor did not induce leukemic lesions, but it did cause a high incidence of nephroblastoma and some cases of visceral lymphomatosis and osteopetrosis.

Nephroblastomas were induced by cell-free extracts of myeloblastosis virus strain A (Beard), and after serial transplantation in chickens. The resulting tumors were studied by electron microscopy.[62] Cytoplasmic and intercellular virus particles were observed in both virus-induced and transplanted nephroblastomas. Three apparent sites of virus particle development were observed: (1) cytoplasmic inclusion bodies of probable mitochondrial origin, (2) cytoplasmic aggregates or viral matrix and, (3) the budding process of cellular membranes. It was concluded that there was no evidence derived from the study that virus particles of variable size in different sites of nephroblastoma cells were related to each other or even to the tumor itself.

A comparative study was made of Rous's sarcoma, visceral lymphomatosis, erythroblastosis, myeloblastosis, and nephroblastoma.[63] Maturation of virus particles by budding of cellular membranes was observed much more frequently in nephroblastoma than in specimens of the other diseases. In addition, the simultaneous presence in single nephroblastoma cells of cytoplasmic inclusions, viral matrix, and budding suggested that virus formation in nephroblastoma proceeded at a much higher rate than in the other chicken neoplasms studied.

In the first of two reports dealing with the multiplicity of cellular response to the BAI strain A virus,[64] the results suggested that infection of nephrogenic cells by virus gives rise to undifferentiated stromal elements from which all other structures of a nephroblastoma are derived. The second report,[65] dealing with the ultrastructure of virus-induced nephroblastoma, suggested that the tumor arises by a series of parallel and discontinuous processes of proliferation and differentiation of primitive nephrogenic elements residual in the postembryonic kidney. Virus was found in the cellular elements of all component tissues of the tumor, and virus release was by budding from the cytoplasmic membrane.

A transmissible nephroblastoma of chickens that contained virions morphologically similar to avian leukosis viruses was inoculated intraperitoneally into 24-hour-old lymphomatosis-free chicks.[66] Two chicks were sacrificed from postinoculation day 2 through day 13, and then at weekly intervals until the seventeenth week. Tissues were examined histologically and by electron microscopy. After 5 to 6 days, virus particles were present in the bone marrow and also in the intracellular spaces in the spleen, and initial virus production occurred in the main hematopoietic organs for 3 to 5 weeks, after which it became quite low. After 10 to 12 days postinoculation, viral particles were found in the visceral organs. Viral particles were observed in kidney tissues only 25 days postinoculation, and only the kidney underwent malignant transformation.

Chemicals

Renal neoplasms up to 4 cm in diameter were found in rainbow trout continuously fed diethylnitrosamine (DMN) for 12 to 20 months.[67] Other trout, 6 months old, were given 1 or 5 intraperitoneal injections each of $100/\mu C$ of I^{131} and raised on an iodine-free diet for up to 24 months; these trout also developed renal tumors. The DMN-induced tumors were less well differentiated than were I^{131}-induced tumors. All of 13 neoplasms examined histologically were characterized by poorly differentiated or anomalous glomeruli and renal tubules interspersed with reticular and collagenous interstitial tissue of variable amounts. Nephroblastomas also developed in rats fed DMN.[68]

Nine transplantable nephroblastomas were established from tumors induced in

Fisher and Sprague-Dawley rats by injecting cycasin or feeding the aglycone of cycasin.[69] Seven of the tumors were successfully transplanted by the intraperitoneal route for 3 to 7 generations. In several nephroblastoma lines, tumors transplanted into the opposite sex from that of the original animal either did not take or grew more slowly than those transplanted to animals of the same sex. Several nephroblastomas were faster-growing in early transfer generations, during which time sex dependency disappeared. Nephroblastomas also were induced in Wistar rats fed cycasin, and the author suggested that nephroblastomas be considered primary mixed tumors.[70]

Intact and ovariectomized female Sprague-Dawley rats 50 days old were given 7,12-dimethylbenzanthracene via intragastric tube.[71] There was an 80% decrease in the incidence of mammary tumor in the ovariectomized rats, but nephroblastomas appeared in 14% of the castrated females between the fifth and eighth months. None occurred in the intact rats.

Nephroblastomas were induced in Wistar rats by feeding nitrosomethyl-urea.[72] The tumors were studied histologically, histochemically, by electron microscopy, and by histoautoradiography. The histologic picture and enzyme composition corresponded to renal tubules. By electron microscopy, a partially retained brush border was seen, the cells of which had a tritiated thymidine index (i.e., the ratio of tumor cells showing incorporation of radioactive thymidine versus incorporation of the isotope by adjacent tumor-free cells) of 1.4% compared to 0.2% for tumor-free areas of the kidney. Undifferentiated epithelial cells also were observed that were rich in ribosomes, and the tritiated thymidine index of these cells was as high as 25%. It was not determined whether these latter cells were carcinogen-induced or were simply hyperplastic cells.

Azoxymethane was given by single subcutaneous injection to BD rats at 1, 3, 10, 30, and 60 days of age, and to adult rats.[73] Of 220 treated rats 29% developed nephroblastomas when the chemical was given at from 1 to 60 days of age, indicating that development of this tumor was not age-dependent.

RESULTS OBTAINED IN *IN VITRO* INVESTIGATIONS OF WILMS' TUMOR AND NEPHROBLASTOMAS OF LOWER ANIMALS

Available Cell Cultures of Wilms' Tumor

Seven cell culture seed stocks of Wilms' tumor are currently available. Six of the seven cultures, in low passage, are listed in the 1974 catalog issued by the Cell Culture Division of the Biomedical Research Laboratory.[74] The other Wilms' tumor cell culture may be obtained from the American Type Collection (ATTC) as TuWi, CCL-31 at approximately the fifty-third cell culture passage.[75]

Cultivation of Wilms' Tumor in Cell Culture

Foley, et al.[76] described the successful isolation and serial propagation in cell culture of normal and malignant tissues from humans and animals in a modified Eagle's basal medium containing calf serum and m-inositol. One of the cell cultures (CCRF-6) was derived from a surgically removed Wilms' tumor.

It was the objective of an investigation in Russia[77] to establish long-term cell cultures from certain human tumors. One of the cell cultures which had been maintained for 1 year was explanted from a Wilms' tumor. This cell culture is epithelioid in appearance, and is the TuWi culture presently available from ATCC.

McAllister, et al.[78] attempted to unmask viruses from human neoplastic and nonneoplastic tissues, employing long-term cultures of small biopsy specimens. Of 6 Wilms' tumors which they cultivated in cell culture, 3 yielded circular or elongated cells containing from 3 to 10 nuclei. Similar cells were not observed in histopathologic sections. Although these results suggested the possibility of still unmasked viruses in the cell cultures, no viruses were clearly demonstrated.

Among 21 primary and metastatic tumors of human kidney and bladder explanted to cell culture, 1 was a Wilms' tumor that was successfully subcultured 14 times during a period of 9 months.[79] No further characterization of this cell culture was mentioned.

The cultivation of a Wilms' tumor in cell culture was reported[80] that appeared fibroblastoid during the first 24 passages. The cells gradually underwent a transition to an epithelioid type beginning with the twenty-fifth passage, and was the predominant cell type at the thirty-first subculture. There was no evidence of the presence of virus particles at this passage level. Growth medium from the fortieth subculture was subjected to centrifugation at 105,000 g and the pellet was sectioned and examined by electron microscopy (EM). Viruslike particles 45 to 50 $m\mu$ in diameter were observed. Ultrathin sections of subsequent cell passages examined by EM revealed viruslike particles in both nucleus and cytoplasm. All attempts to demonstrate virus from this Wilms' tumor cell culture by in vitro and in vivo methods were unsuccessful.

We have had experience in this laboratory with 2 Wilms' tumor cell cultures (unpublished), TE0088 from the Cell Culture Division of the Biomedical Research Laboratory and TuWi from ATCC. Most of our results were obtained with the TE0088 culture, which derived from a 1-year-old male. This cell culture was mixoploid, with chromosome counts ranging from subdiploid to tetraploid (Figure 3). There was an approximate 5% incidence of endoreduplicated cells in the near-diploid range (Figure 4). The diploid cells (Figure 5) were truly diploid both in chromosome number (46) and karyotype (44 + XY). This cell culture was exposed with four animal viruses, vesicular stomatitis virus, parainfluenza virus, type 3, pseudorabies virus, and Newcastle disease virus. All of these viruses were

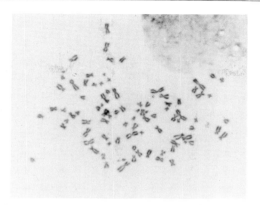

Figure 3. Metaphase spread of a tetraploid (92 chromosomes) cell from the tenth passage of the TE0088 Wilms' tumor cell culture. (Giemsa stain, ×890.)

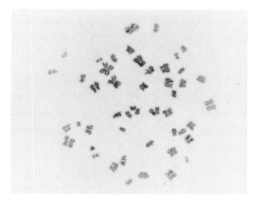

Figure 4. Metaphase spread of an endoreduplicated diploid cell from the tenth passage of the TE0088 Wilms' tumor cell culture. (Giemsa stain, ×890.)

cytopathogenic for the TE0088 cell culture (Figure 6a–6e). Dobrynin et al.[81] reported that their TuWi cell culture formed a compact single layer of epithelioid cells with limited multilayer cellular foci, and that cytogenetic studies revealed a modal number of 60. Our own results with the TuWi culture are in general agreement with Dobrynin's. Our findings indicate that the cells in monolayers of TuWi cultures have very scant cytoplasm, and that they are composed of heteroploid cells with chromosome counts ranging from 49 to 153, with a clustering of cells in the 61 to 64 range.

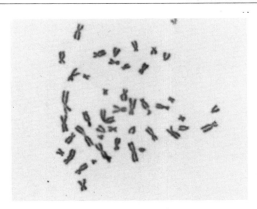

Figure 5.   Metaphase spread of a diploid (46 chromosomes) cell from the tenth passage of the TE0088 Wilms' tumor cell culture. (Giemsa stain, ×1170.)

Chromosome Constitution of Wilms' Tumors With and Without Short-Term Culturing

Direct chromosome analyses, without preliminary tissue culture, were carried out on 7 primary, untreated Wilms' tumors.[82] Of the tumors, 4 had an abnormal chromosome set in which 1 was pseudodiploid and 3 had a slight degree of aneuploidy. The 3 remaining tumors appeared to be typically diploid both in chromosome number and karyotype.

In one[83] of two reports, Rousseau presented the results of chromosome studies of two Wilms' tumors after short-term culture. In one culture there was diploidy with a slight tendency toward polyploidy, and the second culture had aneuploidy with a homogenous distribution of mitoses with a mode of 53. In the second report,[84] results are presented of chromosome analyses of 20 embryonal tumors, 6 of which were Wilms' tumors. Numerical and structural abnormalities were observed in 11 cases, most of which were embryonal sarcomas. Chromosomal abnormalities were less common in the Wilms' tumors, and structural abnormalities were rare.

Growth Promotion *in vitro* by Extracts from Wilms' Tumor

A protein-polysaccharide complex, extracted from a Wilms' tumor or serum from Wilms' tumor-bearing children by acidification with 3% acetic acid, enhanced the proliferation of human embryonic kidney (HEK) cell cultures.[85] The extracts also enhanced the growth of both primary and continuous diploid HEK and lung cell lines. The authors conjecture that the protein-polysaccharide from Wilms' tumor or serum is involved in metastasis by acting as a carrier for malignant cells by assisting them to enlodge at metastatic loci, and aiding in the proliferation of malignant cells once they are established at new loci.

Laboratory Basis for Treatment of Wilms' Tumor

The Furth rat nephroblastoma, which resembles Wilms' tumor histologically and which consistently metastasizes to the lung, was used to assess the best course of clinical treatment of Wilms' tumor.[86] Using the rat tumor model, actinomycin D, vincristine, and X-irradiation were each used alone or in combination to determine the effects on the tumor cells in culture, or on tumors in the rat. The results of both the *in vitro* and *in vivo* experiments indicated that of various combinations, actinomycin D plus X-irradiation proved to be the most effective treatment in killing cells and for rat survival. The nephroblastoma induced in testicular tissue of inbred 129/SV mice by transplanting fetal renal blastema was most effectively arrested by a combination of actinomycin D and vincristine sulfate.[60]

Cell Cultures of Nephroblastomas of Lower Animals

A stable cell line of rat nephroblastoma was initiated from the thirteenth rat passage of the tumor.[87] After more than 5 years in culture, the monolayer was composed of a mixture of spindle-shaped and polygonal cells. Cultured cells were readily transplantable to young Wistar rats by inoculating 1,000,000 or more cells subcutaneously or intraperitoneally. The transplants often regressed spontaneously.

In 1970 we reported the *in vitro* cultivation and characterization of two swine nephroblastoma cell lines.[88] The progress of the primary culture of the first explanted tumor from 3 hours through 5 days is shown in Figures 7a to 7d. It will be noted that the monolayer was composed of epithelioid cells and that contact inhibition of cell growth was pronounced. First passage subcultures of both cell lines were diploid, but both cultures gradually became aneuploid around a mode of 38 chromosomes (diploid for domesticated swine). Cloning efficiencies of both cell lines increased during 45 subcultures and reached 50% in one of the cultures. Primary cell cultures of the first tumor did not induce neoplasia in the cheek pouch of unconditioned Syrian hamsters during a 60-day period after inoculation of 900,000 cells. Likewise, primary cell cultures of the second tumor failed to induce neoplasia in 6-day-old specific pathogen-free pigs during a 30-day observation period after inoculation of 700,000 cells subcutaneously, or after intraperitoneal inoculation of 1,400,000 cells.

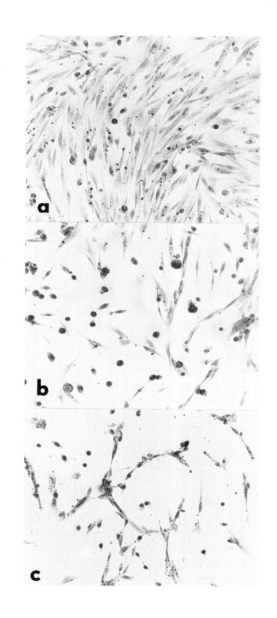

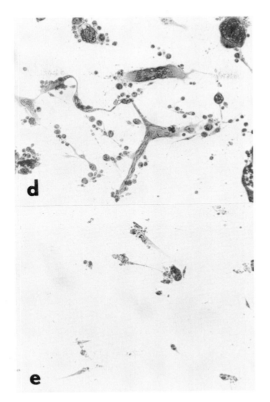

Figure 6. Cytopathic effect (CPE) of four animal viruses in the TE0088 Wilms' tumor cell culture. (Giemsa stain, ×125.) *(a)* Uninoculated monolayer of TE0088 cell culture. *(b)* The CPE produced by vesicular stomatitis virus. *(c)* The CPE produced by parainfluenza type 3 virus. *(d)* The CPE produced by pseudorabies virus. *(e)* The CPE produced by Newcastle disease virus.

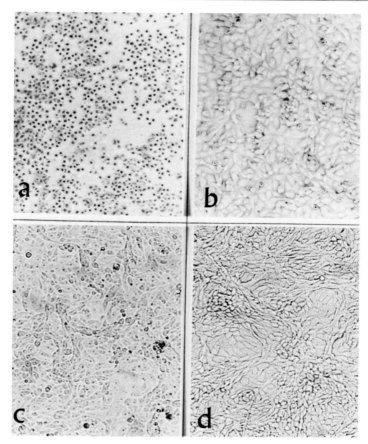

Figure 7.   Progress of a primary cell culture of a swine nephroblastoma from 3 hours through 120 hours of incubation. (Unstained, ×205.) *(a) 3 hours after initial seeding. (b)* 22 hours after seeding. *(c)* 46 hours after seeding. *(d)* 120 hours after seeding. (Reprinted with permission of the *American Journal of Veterinary Research.* [88])

SUMMARY

Spontaneous nephroblastomas of embryonal origin, which are histologically related to Wilms' tumor in humans, occur in a wide range of mammalian species and also in other lower animals. Nephroblastomas of animal species have a much lower potentiality for metastasizing when compared to Wilms' tumor in humans. Regardless of the species in which nephroblastoma occurs spontaneously, all elements of the tumor arise from primitive nephrogenic blastema of mesodermal origin.

Nephroblastomas can be induced in animals experimentally by transplantation of fetal renal blastema, by transplantation of tumor elements, by inoculation with viruses of the avian leukosis complex, and by feeding or inoculating a variety of chemicals.

Wilms' tumor of humans and nephroblastomas of lower animals can be successfully explanted to grow in cell culture *in vitro*. Human and animal nephroblastomas may be essentially diploid in early passages in cell culture, but become aneuploid with continued subculturing.

ACKNOWLEDGMENTS

The author is indeed grateful to Mrs. Helen Hill for literature retrieval; to Dr. Dale Ball, federal meat inspector, Perry, Iowa, for providing the swine nephroblastoma depicted photographically in this chapter; to Dr. Harley Moon, of the National Animal Disease Center, for his expertise in pathology; and to the photographic section of our laboratory.

REFERENCES

1. Wilms, Max: Die Mischgeschwülste der Niere. In *Die Mischgeschwülste*, A. Georgi, Leipzig, Germany, 1899.
2. Lee-Tsun, H., and Holman, R. L.: Bilateral nephroblastoma in a premature infant. *J. Pathol. Bacteriol.* **82**:249–255, 1961.
3. Moulton, J. E.:*Tumors in Domestic Animals*, University of California Press, Berkeley, 1961, pp. 148–151.
4. Jubb, K. V. F., and Kennedy, P. C.:*Pathology of Domestic Animals*, (Vol. 2), Academic Press, New York, 1970, pp. 316–318.
5. Robbins, S. L.: *Textbook of Pathology*, W. B. Saunders Company, Philadelphia, 1957, pp. 940–941.
6. Willis, R. A.: *Pathology of Tumours*, 3rd ed., Butterworth, Washington, D.C., 1960, pp. 929–943.
7. Feldman, W. H.: *Neoplasms of Domesticated Animals*, W. B. Saunders Company, Philadelphia, 1932, pp. 357–372.
8. Sullivan, D. J., and Anderson, W. A.: Embryonal nephroma in swine. *Am. J. Vet. Res.* **20**:324–332, 1959.
9. Migaki, G., Nelson, L. W., and Todd, G. C.: Prevalence of embryonal nephroma in slaughtered swine. *J. Am. Vet. Med. Assoc.* **159**:441–442, 1971.
10. Cotchin, E.: Tumours of farm animals; a survey of tumours examined at the royal veterinary college, London, during 1950–1960. *Vet. Rec.* **72**:816–822, 1960.

11. Sandison, A. T., and Anderson, L. J.: Tumors of the kidney in cattle, sheep and pigs. *Cancer* **21**:727–742, 1968.

12. Kataria, R. S., and Soni, J. L.: Porcine nephroblastoma. *Indian Vet. J.* **44**:555–557, 1967.

13. Feldman, W. H., and Olson, C.: Neoplastic diseases of the chicken. In Biester, H. E., and Schwarte, L. H., (Eds.: *Diseases of Poultry*, (5th ed.), Iowa State University Press, Ames, 1965, pp. 913–924.

14. Feldman, W. H., and Olson, C.: Keratinizing embryonal nephroma of the kidneys of the chicken. *Am. J. Cancer* **19**:47–55, 1933.

15. McKenney, F. D.: Embryonal nephroma in the chicken: report of two cases. *Am. J. Cancer* **15**:122–128, 1931.

16. Helmboldt, C. F., and Fredrickson, T. N.: The avian leukosis complex. In *Comparative Morphology of Hematopoietic Neoplasms, Natl. Cancer Inst. Monogr.* **32**:29–42, 1969.

17. Mathews, F. P.: Adenosarcomata of the kidneys of chickens. *J. Am. Vet. Med. Assoc.* **74**:238–246, 1929.

18. Krishnan, R.: A note on an embryonal nephroma met with in a fowl. *Indian Vet. J.* **46**:286–288, 1969.

19. Walker, R.: Embryonal nephroma in a calf. *J. Am. Vet. Med. Assoc.* **102**:7–10, 1943.

20. Misdorp, W.: Tumours in newborn animals. *Pathol. Vet.* **2**:328–343, 1965.

21. Kirkbride, C. A., and Bicknell, E. J.: Nephroblastoma in a bovine fetus. *Vet. Pathol.* **9**:96–98, 1972.

22. Bullock, F. D., and Curtis, M. R.: Spontaneous tumors of the rat. *J. Cancer Res.* **14**:1–115, 1930.

23. Hottendorf, G. H., and Ingraham, K. J.: Spontaneous nephroblastomas in laboratory rats. *J. Am. Vet. Med. Assoc.* **153**:826–829, 1968.

24. Magnusson, G.: Spontaneous nephroblastomas in the rat. *Z. Versuchstierk.* **11**:293–297, 1969.

25. Gohlke, R., and Schmidt, P.: Spontanes Ratten-Nephroblastom. *Z. Versuchstierk.* **13**:326–337, 1971.

26. Pittermann, W.: Spontane nephroblastome bei SPF-Ratten. *Berl. Munch. Tierarztl. Worchenschr.* **87**:58, 1974.

27. Weitz, W. L., and McClelland, R. B.: Embryonal nephroma in a dog. *J. Am. Vet. Med. Assoc.* **97**:604–605, 1940.

28. Drew, R. A., Done, S. H., and Robins, G. M.: Canine embryonal nephroma; a case report. *J. Small Anim. Pract.* **13**:27–39, 1972.

29. Coleman, G. L., Gralla, E. J., Knirsch, A. K., and Stebbins, R. B.: Canine embryonal nephroma; a case report. *Am. J. Vet. Res.* **31**:1315–1320, 1970.

30. Sagartz, J. W., Ayers, K. M., Cashell, I. G., and Robinson, F. R.: Malignant embryonal nephroma in an aged dog. *J. Am. Vet. Med. Assoc.* **161**:1658–1660, 1972.

31. Fiedler, H. H., and Redecker, R.: Embyonales Nephrom bei einem zenjahrigen Hund. *Dtsch. Tierarztl. Wochenschr.* **80**:458–459, 1973.

32. Bell, E. T., and Henrici, A. T.: Renal tumors in the rabbit. *J. Cancer Res.* **1**:157–167, 1916.

33. Scott, E.: Tumors of the kidney in rabbits. *J. Cancer Res.* **2**:367–371, 1917.

34. Greene, H. S. N.: The occurrence and transplantations of embryonal nephromas in the rabbit. *Cancer Res.* **3**:434–440, 1943.

35. Potkay, S., and Garman, R.: Nephroblastoma in a cat; the effects of nephrectomy and occlusion of the caudal vena cava. *J. Small Anim. Pract.* **10**:345–349, 1969.

36. Kharole, M. U., and Rao, U. R. K.: Embryonal nephroma in goats. *Indian Vet. J.* **49**:1086–1089, 1972.

37. Feldman, W. H.: Embryonal nephroma in a sheep. *Am. J. Cancer* **17**:743–747, 1933.

38. Herman, L. H.: Embryonal nephroma in a parakeet. *Vet. Med.* **64**:812–813, 1969.

39. Zwart, P.: A nephroblastoma in a fire-bellied newt, *Cynops pyrrhogaster. Cancer Res.* **30**:2691–2694, 1970.

40. Helmboldt, C. F., and Wyand, D. S.: Nephroma in a striped bass. *J. Wildlife Dis.* **7**:162–165, 1971.

41. Toolan, H. W.: The growth of human tumors in cortisone-treated laboratory animals; the possibility of obtaining permanently transplantable human tumors. *Cancer Res.* **13**:389–394, 1953.

42. Toolan, H. W.: Transplantable human neoplasms maintained in cortisone-treated laboratory animals: HS#1, HEp#1, HEp#2, HEp#3, and HEmbRh#1. *Cancer Res.* **14**:660–666, 1954.

43. Olcott, C. T.: A transplantable nephroblastoma (Wilms' tumor) and other spontaneous tumors in a colony of rats. *Cancer Res.* **10**:625–628, 1950.

44. Babcock, V. I., and Southam, C. M.: Transplantable renal tumor of the rat. *Cancer Res.* **21**:130–134, 1961.

45. Tomashefsky, P., Furth, J., Lattimer, J. K., et al.: The Furth-Columbia rat Wilms' tumor. *J. Urol.* **107**:348–354, 1972.

46. Adler, S., and Theodor, O.: Investigations on Meditteranean kala azar. I. Introduction and epidemiology. *Proc. Roy. Soc., B.* **108**:447–453, 1931.

47. Adler, S.: Origin of the golden hamster *Cricetus auratus* as a laboratory animal. *Nature (Lond.)* **162**:256–257, 1948.

48. Lutz, B. R., Fulton, G. P., Patt, D. I., and Handler, A. H.: The growth rate of tumor transplants in the cheek pouch of the hamster. *Cancer Res.* **10**:231–232, 1950.

49. Lutz, B. R., Fulton, G. P., Patt, D. I., et al.: The cheek pouch of the hamster as a site for the transplantation of a methyl-cholanthrene-induced sarcoma. *Cancer Res.* **11**:64–67, 1951.

50. Handler, A. H., Patt, D. I., and Lutz, B. R.: Growth of heterologous tumors in the hamster cheek pouch. *Anat. Rec.* **112**:449–450, 1952.

51. Chute, R. N., Sommers, S. C., and Warren, S.: Heterotransplantation of human cancer. II. Hamster cheek pouch. *Cancer Res.* **12**:912–914, 1952.

52. Patterson, W. B., Chute, R. N., and Sommers, S. C.: Transplantation of human tumors into cortisone-treated hamsters. *Cancer Res.* **14**:656–659, 1954.

53. Handler, A. H., Davis, S., and Sommers, S. C.: Heterotransplantation experiments with human cancer. *Cancer Res.* **16**:32–36, 1956.

54. Handler, A. H., and Foley, G. E.: Growth of human epidermoid carcinomas (strains KB and HeLa) in hamsters from tissue culture inoculua. *Proc. Soc. Exp. Biol. Med.* **91**:237–240, 1956.

55. Handler, A. H.: Growth of tumors from children in the cheek pouch of the golden hamster. *Proc. Am. Assoc. Cancer Res.* **2**:114, 1956.

56. Handler, A. H.: Chemotherapy studies on transplantable human and animal tumors in Syrian hamsters. *Ann. N.Y. Acad. Sci.* **76**:775–790, 1958.

57. Foley, G. E., and Handler, A. H.: Differentiation of "normal" and neoplastic cells maintained in tissue culture by implantation into normal hamsters. *Proc. Soc. Exp. Biol. Med.* **94**:661–664, 1957.

58. Foley, G. E., Handler, A. H., Adams, R. A. and Craig, J. M.: Assessment of potential

malignancy of cultured cells: Further observations on the differentiation of "normal" and "neoplastic" cells maintained *in vitro* by heterotransplantation in Syrian hamsters. *Natl. Cancer Inst. Monogr.* 7:173–204, 1962.

59. Foley, G. E., and Handler, A. H.: Tumorigenic activity of tissue cell cultures. *Ann. N.Y. Acad. Sci.* 76:506–512, 1958.

60. Javadpour, N., and Bush, I. M.: Induction and treatment of Wilms' tumor by transplantation of renal blastema in a new experimental model. *J. Urol.* 107:931–937, 1972.

61. Walter, W. G., Burmester, B. R., and Cunningham, C. H.: Studies on the transmission and pathology of a viral-induced avian nephroblastoma (embryonal nephroma). *Avian Dis.* 6:455–477, 1962.

62. Dmochowski, L., Grey, C. E., Burmester, B. R., and Walter, W. G.: Submicroscopic morphology of avian neoplasms. V. Studies on nephroblastoma. *Texas Rep. Biol. Med.* 19:545–579, 1961.

63. Dmochowski, L., Grey, C. E., Padgett, F., Langford, P. L., and Burmester, B. R.: Submicroscopic morphology of avian neoplasms. VI. Comparative studies of Rous sarcoma, visceral lymphomatosis, erythroblastosis, myeloblastosis, and nephroblastoma. *Texas Rep. Biol. Med.* 22:20–60, 1964.

64. Ishiguro, H., Beard, D., Sommer, J. R., et al.: Multiplicity of cell response to the BAI strain A (myeloblastosis) avian tumor virus. I. Nephroblastoma (Wilms' tumor); gross and microscopic pathology. *J. Natl. Cancer Inst.* 29:1–39, 1962.

65. Heine, U., de Thé, G., Ishiguro, H., et al.: Multiplicity of cell response to the BAI strain A (myeloblastosis) avian tumor virus. II. Nephroblastoma (Wilms' tumor); ultrastructure. *J. Natl. Cancer Inst.* 29:41–105, 1962.

66. Weiler, O., Delain, E., and Lacour, F.: Studies on a viral nephroblastic nephroblastoma of the chicken: an electron microscope comparison of the sequence of development of the virions in different organs. *Eur. J. Cancer* 7:491–494, 1971.

67. Ashley, L. M.: Renal neoplasms of rainbow trout. *Bull. Wildl. Dis. Assoc.* 3:86 (abstr.), 1967.

68. Hadjiolov, D.: Induction of nephroblastomas in the rat with dimethylnitrosamine. *Z. Krebsforsch.* 71:59–62, 1968.

69. Hirono, I., Laqueur, G. L., and Spatz, M.: Transplantability of cycasin-induced tumors in rats, with emphasis on nephroblastomas. *J. Natl. Cancer Inst.* 40:1011–1025, 1968.

70. Gusek, W.: Feinstruktur und differenzierung experimenteller Wilmstumoren. *Verh. Dtsch. Ges. Pathol.* 52:410–415, 1968.

71. Jasmin, G., and Riopelle, J. I.: Nephroblastomas induced in ovariectomized rats by dimethylbenzanthracene. *Cancer Res.* 30:321–326, 1970.

72. Thomas, C., Wessel, W., and Citoler, P.: Histochemische, elektronenmikroskopische und autoradiographische Untersuchungen an experimentell erzeugten Nephroblastomen. *Beitr. Pathol.* 145:68–82, 1972.

73. Druckrey, H., and Lange, A.: Carcinogenicity of azoxymethane dependent on age in BD rats. *Fed. Proc.* 31:1482–1484, 1972.

74. *Catalog of human and other animal cell cultures.* Cell Culture Laboratory, University of California, School of Public Health, Naval Biomedical Research Laboratory, Naval Supply Center, Oakland, September, 1974.

75. *Registry of Animal Cell Lines Certified by the Cell Culture Collection Committee*, (2nd ed.), American Type Culture Collection Cell Repository, Rockville, Md., 1972.

76. Foley, G. E., Drolet, B. P., McCarthy, R. E., et al.: Isolation and serial propagation of

malignant and normal cells in semi-defined media; origins of CCRF cell lines. *Cancer Res.* **20**:930–939, 1960.

77. Dobrynin, Y. V.: Establishment and characteristics of cell strains from some epithelial tumors of human origin. *J. Natl. Cancer Inst.* **31**:1173–1195, 1963.

78. McAllister, R. M., Mikenas, M., Straw, R. M., and Landing, B. H.: Cytologic and virologic studies of cultures derived from neoplastic and non-neoplastic tissues of children. *Lab. Invest.* **12**:342–354, 1963.

79. Jones, G. W.: Primary and metastatic epithelial tumors of the human kidney and bladder in tissue culture. *Cancer* **20**:1893–1898, 1967.

80. Smith, J. W., Pinkel, C., and Dabrowski, S.: Detection of a small virus in a cultivated human Wilms' tumor. *Cancer* **24**:527–531, 1969.

81. Dobrynin, Y. V., Obukhova, L. E., and Mirzoyan, E. E.: Kharakteristika linii kletok opukholi vil'msa in vitro. *Vopr. Onkol.* **12**:30–38, 1966.

82 Cox, D.: Chromosome constitution of nephroblastomas. *Cancer* **19**:1217–1224, 1966.

83. Rousseau, M. F., Laurent M., and Nezelof, C.: Le nephroblastome; Etude chromosomique. *Ann. Anat. Pathol. (Paris)* **15**:399–414, 1970.

84. Rousseau, M. F.: Etude chromosomique de 20 tumeurs embryonaries apres culture a court terme. *Biomed. Express (Paris)* **19**:275–280, 1973.

85. Beierle, J. W., Heimerl, D. M., Allerton, S. E., and Bavetta, L. A.: Growth promotion by extracts from Wilms' tumor in vitro. *Experientia* **27**:435–436, 1971.

86. Priestley, J. B.: The laboratory basis for the clinical treatment of Wilms' tumor. *J. Urol.* **107**:696–704, 1972.

87. Babcock, V. I., and Southam, C. M.: Stable cell line of rat nephroma in tissue culture. *Proc. Soc. Exp. Biol. Med.* **124**:217–219, 1967.

88. Pirtle, E. C., Mengeling, W. L., and Cheville, N. F.: Initiation and characterization of two porcine embryonal nephroma cell lines. *Am. J. Vet. Res.* **31**:1601–1608, 1970.

CHAPTER SEVEN

Histopathology of Wilms' Tumor and Related Lesions

H. JOACHIM WIGGER, M.D.

Associate Professor of Clinical Pediatric Pathology
College of Physicians and Surgeons
Columbia University
Associate Attending Pathologist
Division of Developmental Pathology
Presbyterian Hospital
New York, New York

CONTENTS

The histopathology of Wilms' tumor has been well investigated. In fact, light microscopic descriptions have changed little since Wilms' original monograph of 1899.[1] The latest review generally cited is not only more than a decade old, but has also added little more than an arrangement of the recognized histologic patterns in a classification.[2] Chapters on Wilms' tumor in standard textbooks of pathology reflect the lack of new information and concepts over a period of many years;[3-7] at times pathologic descriptions have been transferred from older editions almost verbatim.[5] The significance of histologic features in relation to prognosis of the patient has either not been mentioned or has been denied.[3-6,8-10] It is, therefore, not surprising that at present the value of histologic features for the clinician does not extend beyond their use in substantiating the diagnosis of Wilms' tumor.

During recent years it has become apparent that variations in histologic composition and differentiation have a bearing on the prognosis in addition to the clinical and pathologic stage of the disease and the nature of the initial therapy. This implies that the histologic type may directly influence the progression of the disease and thus its stage. In cases of identical stage and initial therapy, the outcome may depend primarily on the histologic type. Therefore these histologic features may even be more important prognostic indicators than many factors thought to be significant thus far.[8-15] It is such evidence that makes a new look at the histopathology of Wilms' tumor necessary and applicable to clinical management.

WILMS' TUMOR

The clinical picture of malignant renal tumors in infancy and childhood was already known in the late eighteenth century.[2] It was, however, not until the last third of the nineteenth century that an understanding of their nature resulted from investigations with newly acquired techniques and knowledge of pathologic anatomy.

In this period, the first reports were impressed with the prominence of skeletal muscle in these tumors.[16,17] Their possible bilaterality was recognized by Hansen in 1873,[18] and two years later Strum[19] commented on their mixed sarcomatous and epithelial composition. Birch-Hirschfeld[20] placed emphasis on the blastemal ("archiblastische") elements and suggested the term embryonal adenosarcoma to reflect the mixed and immature composition of the tumor. Max Wilms reviewed the experience with pediatric renal tumors in his monograph of 1899.[1] Although some reports preceded his publication, Wilms must be credited with the first detailed review and interpretation of these tumors. He agreed with Cohnheim[17] that they were probably mesodermal in origin. This hypothesis best explained the mixed composition of these tumors which contain not only undifferentiated blastemal and epithelial elements, but may also contain a large variety of connective tissue components of varying quantity, such as skeletal muscle, myxoid, adipose and fibrous tissue, cartilage and bone.

Wilms' name became firmly associated with these tumors, especially in North America. More descriptive terms, such as embryoma or embryonal adenosarcoma, fell into disuse after McCurdy introduced the name nephroblastoma, now used synonymously with the eponym.[21] Culp and Hartmann suggested mesoblastic nephroma to recall the mesodermal derivation of the tumor, but this term never became popular.[22]

Histologic Classification of Wilms' Tumor

For the most part, periodic reviews of Wilms' tumor pathology restated previous descriptions.[2, 23-26] Bodian and Rigby[2] proposed a histologic classification which reflects the variability of the tumor both in terms of tissue composition and tissue differentiation or maturity. According to this classification, Wilms' tumors are separated into seven types. Some of these histologic types are shown in Figures 1,2, and 3. (A tumor with both benign and malignant elements should be considered a malignant tumor.) Distribution of their cases into these categories resulted in two conclusions: first, a tendency of the more differentiated tumors (types a to d) to occur in the first three years of life; and, secondly, a higher survival in the younger age groups with more differentiated elements. The significance of these conclusions suffered, however, from a low numerical representation of the differentiated tumors. Stowens[27] arrived at conclusions similar to those of Bodian and Rigby from a similarly detailed classification. Subsequent reviewers,[28,29] however, considered the histologic types of little or no consequence to the prognosis. In fact, size or volume of Wilms' tumor seemed to have a much greater bearing on survival.[30,31]

During the last few decades the literature on Wilms' tumor was primarily concerned with therapeutic aspects; recently, however, isolated communications again attempted to derive prognostic indicators from the histologic type. Simplification of the histologic classification, using only degrees of tissue differentiation or maturity, was employed by Stowens.[27] Later studies that followed this example concluded that the more differentiated tumors with large structural components mimicking embryonal kidney had a better prognosis than the less differentiated ones.[12,31,32] In these studies, histologic grading was the only factor assessed.

Jereb and Sandstedt[11] conducted a statistical analysis to evaluate any appreciable interaction among a number of factors which might all have had a bearing on cure and survival. These factors included the patient's age, clinical stage of the disease, tumor size, and histologic type. Since they might influence each other and the cure rate, their separate analysis could conceivably indicate a strong

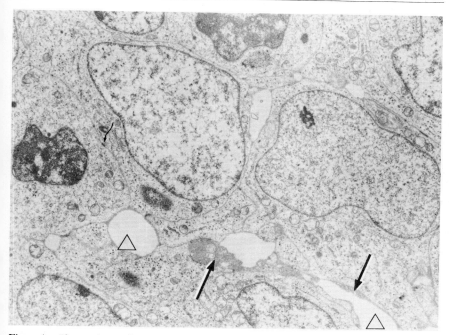

Figure 4. Blastemal type of Wilms' tumor with closely packed cells containing irregular nuclei. The cytoplasm has scant organelles but many polyribosomes. Despite the lack of cellular differentiation, there are basement membrane formations as thin layers or clumps (straight arrow), occasional junctional complexes (curved arrow), and formation of small spaces (open triangle) in the absence of cell polarization, indicating the epithelial nature of the tumor cells. (E.M. 6232.00×).

complexes, luminal polarity of cells, basement membrane formation, and narrow but patent lumina lined with microvilli or even brush borders. Cilia formation occurs in definitive epithelial cell masses and also in mesenchymal cells (Figure 8). A consistent finding in one study[36] was the presence of paired atypical cisternae. Like the neoplastic epithelial cells of Wilms' tumor, the mesenchymal cells showed all degrees of maturation and differentiation from the primitive cells of secondary mesenchyme to the fully developed connective tissue cells of different types. By ultrastructure, the gradual differentiation to fibroblasts and skeletal muscle cells were demonstrated.[36-39]

The similarity of human Wilms' tumor cells to cells of immature normal kidney was striking. No distinct differences could be detected except for an asynchronous development among individual cytoplasmic organelles.[35]

The light and electron microscopical features of experimentally produced Wilm's tumors are very similar to the human form whether they are

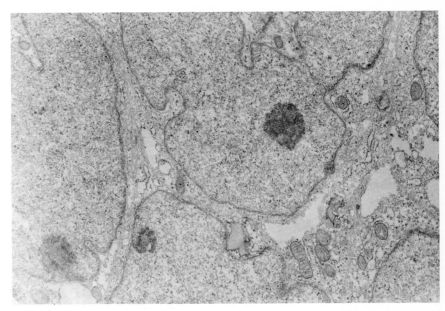

Figure 5. Cells of the tumor in Figure 4 were grown in tissue culture and lost both junctional complexes and basement membranes. (E.M. 8008.00×).

virus-induced,[40,41] cycasin-induced,[42] or spontaneous and transplantable.[43] The only exception is the presence of endothelial cells and capillary lumina in the virus-induced avian nephroblastoma.[41]

VARIANTS OF WILMS' TUMOR

The conventional Wilms' tumor described in the preceding section is composed predominantly of epithelial cells of varying degrees of differentiation and a less prominent connective tissue stromal component. Wilms' tumors predominantly or almost exclusively composed of connective tissue elements are less common. In most of these tumors one connective tissue element stands out (monophasic mesenchymal tumors). It is, however, not only their distinctive histopathology that deserves special attention, but also their different clinical behavior. Perez et al.[12] observed an unexpectedly high survival rate in mesenchymal Wilms' tumors.

Fetal Rhabdomyomatous Nephroblastoma

At the Babies Hospital in New York City, 5 Stage I tumors were studied[15] that were almost entirely composed of fetal skeletal muscle separated by varying amounts of

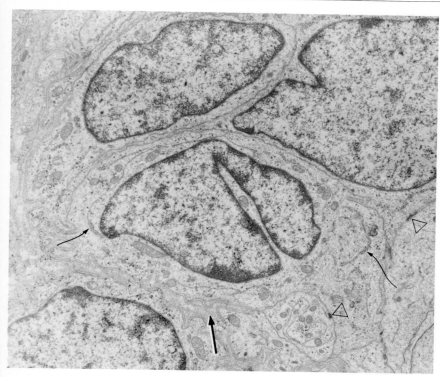

Figure 6. Closely packed Wilms' tumor cells with nuclei showing irregular contour and notching. The cytoplasm contains scant mitochondria and rough endoplasmic reticulum (curved arrow). Basement membrane material is present on parts of the cell surface (straight arrow). Where the plasma membranes are closely opposed, junctional complexes are seen (open triangles). Intricate infoldings simulate the basal surface of tubular epithelial cells (straight arrow). The light microscopy of this case revealed blastemal areas and some tubular differentiation. (See Figure 2.) (E.M. 7866.00×).

mature fibrous tissue. Other connective tissue components were minor. The least mature elements were indistinguishable from metanephric blastema as seen in the embryonal kidney and in Wilms' tumor (Figure 9). There was a gradual transition from these elements to cells that resembled rhabdomyoblasts with scant myofilaments, generally in parallel arrangement, mitochondria and polyribosomes. Z-bands were present in the more differentiated cells (Figures 10,11). The fibrous tissue was composed of mature fibroblasts and collagen. Neoplastic epithelial structures, mostly tubular, were identical to those seen in the conventional Wilms' tumor. The prognosis of these tumors seemed to depend on the amount of this component. A large portion of poorly or moderately differentiated epithelial elements led to abdominal metastases and eventual death in 1 patient. A

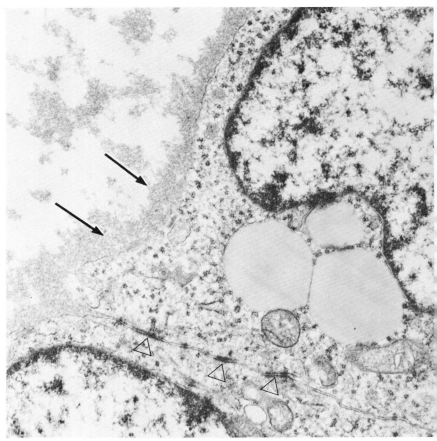

Figure 7. Wilms' tumor epithelial cells with abundant junctional complexes (triangles) and lipid droplets. Ample basement membrane material was laid down (straight arrows). (E.M. 20,160.00×).

small amount was found in 2 patients who were cured by nephrectomy. Local recurrence after incomplete resection developed in 1 case of unilateral tumor, but the patient was free of disease 4 years later. Thus, this case was apparently cured by resection of the recurrence. Bilaterality of one tumor resulted in recurrence on the side of the heminephrectomy and in renal failure. Because of its characteristic microscopic appearance and its relationship to Wilms' tumor, the term fetal rhabdomyomatous nephroblastoma (FRN) was chosen.

This tumor was by no means a recent discovery, since it had been recognized before the conventional Wilms' tumor. About a dozen cases were published before Wilms' monograph appeared in 1899, the classic description being Cohnheim's in

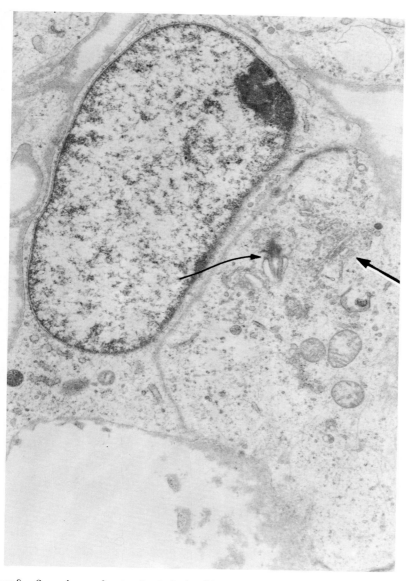

Figure 8. Some degree of maturation is displayed by this Wilms' tumor cell. In addition to thick basement membranes and junctional complexes, distinct Golgi complexes (straight arrow) and basal body of a cilium (curved arrow) appear as well as some degree of polarization of the cell leading to formation of spaces. (E.M. 12,800×).

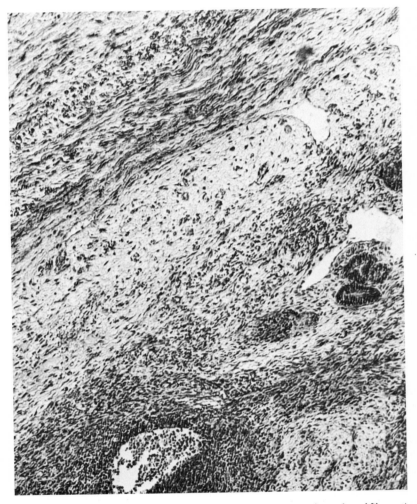

Figure 9. Fetal rhabdomyomatous nephroblastoma (FRN) showing striped muscle and fibrous tissue (upper half) and undifferentiated blastemal and neoplastic tubular elements (lower half). (HPS stain 126×).

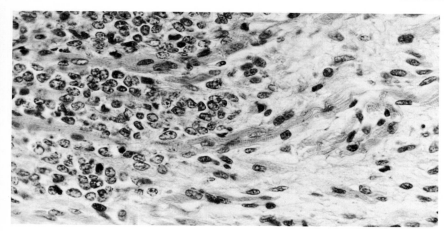

Figure 10.   Transition from immature elements to striated muscle of fetal stage of development in a fetal rhabdomyomatous nephroblastoma. (HPS stain 255×).

1875.[17] Since the conventional Wilms' tumor was also recognized to contain some striated muscle, both lesions were considered closely related and the separate identity of FRN was eventually forgotten.

Fifteen cases from the literature substantiated the findings in the recent cases.[15] Some of the older cases died without any treatment and never showed metastases at autopsy. Of the 15 cases, 3 developed small abdominal metastases; none of the entire group of 20 cases had pulmonary metastases. The FRN were considerably larger than the usual Wilms' tumor (4118 cm³ vs. 380 cm³). The 30% incidence of bilaterality in the FRN was remarkable, more than six times the expected incidence for Wilms' tumor.[44] Clinical and laboratory findings were not diagnostic. None of the cases occurred in patients over 4 years, the average age being 1 year and 8 months.

Osteocartilagenous Nephroblastoma and Lipomatous Nephroblastoma

The almost monophasic growth of striated muscle in FRN raises the question of whether other connective tissue lines may behave in a similar manner. This is indeed the case in adipose[45] and osteocartilaginous[46] tissue, of which one each has been recognized (Figure 12).

HAMARTOMAS

Hamartomas are believed to be faulty mixtures of normal components of an organ either because of a change in quantity, composition, degree of maturation, or all

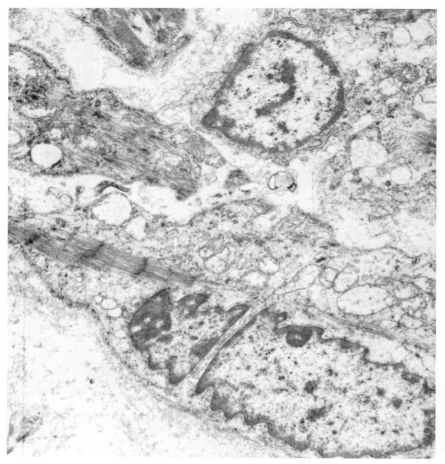

Figure 11.   Immature skeletal muscle cells with scant myofilaments, showing Z-bands. (E.M. 12,000×).

three.[14] They are considered benign and may be related to malformations or neoplasms.[47,48] Lesions may be classified as epithelial hamartomas[14] that are known variously as nephroblastoma in situ,[49] nodular renal blastema,[50] or metanephric hamartoma,[51] and also as nephroblastomatosis.[52]

The best known mesenchymal hamartoma is the angiomyolipoma often associated with tuberous sclerosis. In the differential diagnosis of Wilms' tumor, however, the fetal hamartoma is the only one of importance.[13,14]

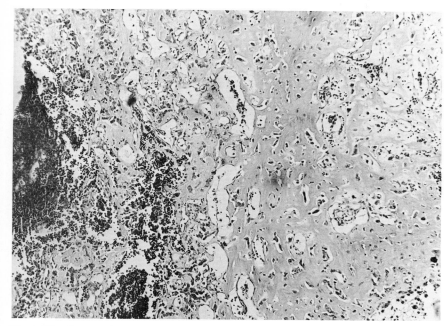

Figure 12. Osteocartilaginous nephroblastoma with blastemal elements (left) and bony and cartilaginous components (right). (HPS stain 80.94×).

Multifocal Epithelial Hamartomas

The multifocal epithelial hamartomas vary in size from microscopic aggregates to small nodules barely visible with the naked eye (Figure 13). Their similarity to Wilms' tumor has led to the designation nephroblastoma in situ,[49] their likeness to metanephric blastema led to the terms nodular renal blastema[50] and metanephric hamartoma.[51] All cases reported by Bove et al.[50] were associated with multiple malformations that were different from those seen in Wilms' tumor. Most of them fell into the group associated with trisomy 18 or closely related to it. In 6 of the 11 cases studied, the abnormal karyotype was confirmed by cytogenetic studies. On the other hand, 5 of 8 cases of trisomy 18 disclosed nodular renal blastema on serial sections of kidney tissue. Epithelial hamartomas and trisomy 18 are frequently observed in females. In contrast, Wilms' tumor patients show a slight preponderance of males, which becomes striking only in combination with aniridia.[53]

The incidence of multifocal epithelial hamartoma is highest in infants under 4 months, 1:400 and 1:235.[49,50] These hamartomas were reported in older patients

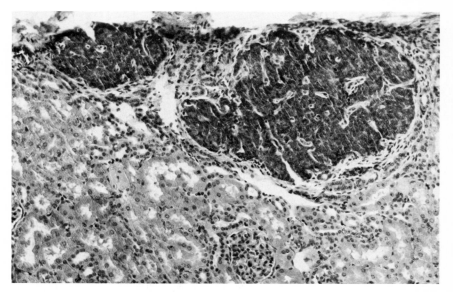

Figure 13. Subcapsular, multifocal epithelial hamartomas (nodular renal blastema) composed of immature blastemal cells. (HPS stain 170.40×).

only in association with Wilms' tumor. Bove et al.[50] noted this in 8 of 46 cases of Wilms' tumor,[5] of which were bilateral. Thus it seems likely that few of these hamartomas are related to Wilms' tumor. The fate of the others is even more uncertain, but histologic evidence suggests that maturation and involution are responsible for the fall in incidence beyond early infancy (Figure 14).

The sudden drop in incidence of multifocal epithelial hamartoma after the age of 4 months corresponds to the experience with neuroblastoma in situ. This lesion has a reported incidence of 1:39 in infants under 6 months,[54] and of 1:179 in infants under 3 months.[55] The expected rate of occurrence for adrenal neuroblastoma lies around 1:10,000.[56,57] The absence of mitoses and the frequency of associated malformations (46%)[54] that are not features of neuroblastoma suggest that the in situ lesion is an unlikely source of neuroblastoma.

Diffuse Epithelial Hamartomas

Bilateral diffuse hamartomas or nephroblastomatosis are rare lesions.[51,52,58-61] They have resulted in renal enlargement with excessive abnormal lobulation. Varying amounts of subcapsular renal cortex were replaced by unencapsulated, immature renal elements. Transition to the normal cortex was either abrupt or gradual (Figure 15). Two of the reported cases were sporadic and not associated

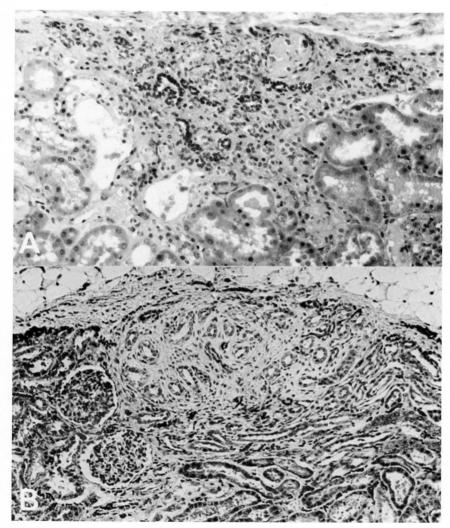

Figure 14. Subcapsular epithelial hamartomas showing degrees of maturation and involution as compared with the lesion in Figure 13. (A. HPS stain 147.20×; B. HPS stain 86.48×).

with malformations; both occurred in premature female infants with cutaneous edema.[52,58] Of 4 term infants reported in a Yemenite Jewish family,[51,60] 2 male infants had multifocal epithelial hamartomas and 2 others had the diffuse type, the female without malformations, the male with multiple congenital anomalies and visceromegaly. The oldest and only surviving patient[61] in this category was a girl

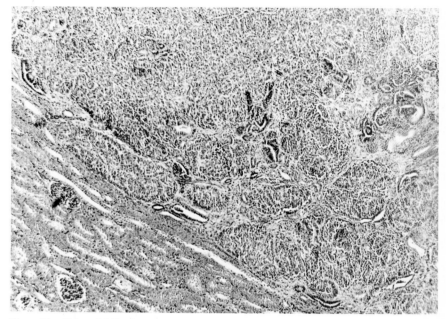

Figure 15.   Bilateral diffuse hamartoma or nephroblastomatosis displays abrupt transition from a zone resembling immature nephrogenic tissue to mature kidney. There is neither compression of the normal kidney parenchyma nor capsule formation, features one could expect with Wilms' tumor. (HPS stain 78.66×).

with Klippel-Trenaunay syndrome, dislocation of the hip, and psychomotor retardation, who underwent nephrectomy for suspected Wilms' tumor before the correct diagnosis was made. The opposite kidney was involved as well but was only biopsied; subsequently radiation therapy and chemotherapy were given. About 6 months postoperatively, a renal biopsy revealed normal renal tissue and disappearance of the originally observed nodularity. This finding suggested at least partial, if not complete, maturation of the lesion.

Fetal Mesenchymal Hamartomas

In some instances this tumor was long considered different from Wilms' tumor and was diagnosed in newborns as spindle cell sarcoma,[62] fibroma,[63] leiomyoma,[64] or leiomyosarcoma.[65] Many were, however, diagnosed as Wilms' tumor. With the introduction of potentially dangerous, aggressive regimens of radiation therapy and chemotherapy it became imperative to determine whether this tumor was malignant. More than 70 such tumors were reported under different names.[66] They all demonstrated remarkably similar clinical and mor-

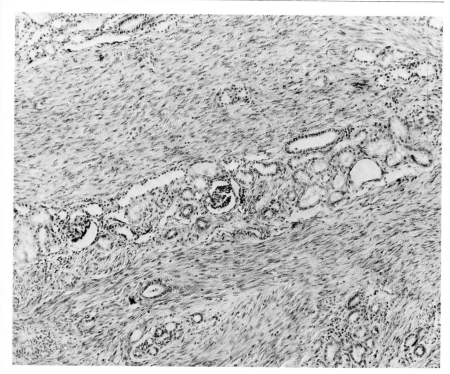

Figure 16. Interlacing bundles of spindle cells in a fetal mesenchymal hamartoma (FMH) grow between normal renal parenchymal elements without compression or destruction. These features suggest growth of the hamartoma at the same, or a slightly faster, rate than the kidney. (HPS stain 95.76×).

phologic features and were all clinically and morphologically different from Wilms' tumor, as pointed out first by Bolande et al.,[13] who called these tumors mesoblastic nephroma. The term fetal mesenchymal hamartoma (FMH) was based on their frequently immature appearance and development during fetal life, on the exclusively mesenchymal character of the tumor, and on the absence of destructive invasiveness and metastases.[14] Local recurrence was observed in 2 cases, but there had been suspicion of residual tumor after the first operation.[67,68] Although grossly well-demarcated, this tumor was not encapsulated like Wilms' tumor; histologically it was not sharply separated from the renal parenchyma, and at times it was not even clearly separated from the perirenal tissues (Figure 16). This does not necessarily imply neoplastic invasion any more than it does in benign hemangioendotheliomas.

Clinical and radiologic features were not helpful in separating FMH from Wilms' tumor. Although FMH probably made up the great majority of neonatal solid tumors of the kidney, Wilms' tumors were also seen in this age group. Thus, histopathologic study provided the only means for accurate differentiation. The interlacing bundles of oval to spindly cells displayed varying degrees of differentiation as demonstrated by nucleocytoplasmic ratio, cell shape, and amount and type of extracellular material. Epithelial elements were included in the tumor, especially adjacent to the kidney. They were considered to represent entrapped normal and also dysplastic, renal parenchymal elements. The absence of neoplastic epithelial structures seemed to be the single most important difference of FMH from Wilms' tumor and was probably responsible for the benign course of fetal mesenchymal hamartoma. [14,69]

High cellularity, frequent mitoses, and inverted nucleocytoplasmic ratio may cause considerable concern about the prospective course in the patient with FMH. The possibility that such immature cells could be epithelial and develop into a Wilms' tumor must be considered. Detailed ultrastructural studies[66] failed to show any cells that could be identified as epithelial. The least mature cells were secondary mesenchymal cells, which differ from primary mesenchymal cells or mesoblasts in that they can produce only connective tissue cells (Figures 17,18). Although different lines of connective tissue could conceivably develop, to date

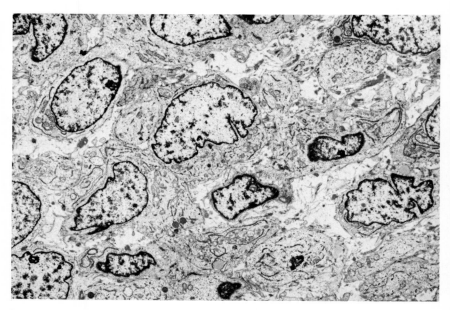

Figure 17. Haphazardly arranged cells of an undifferentiated FMH exhibit irregular nuclei, moderate numbers of cytoplasmic organelles, mostly long profiles of rough endoplasmic reticulum, mitochondria, lipid vacuoles, occasional lysosomes, and microbodies. (E.M. 3,969.00×).

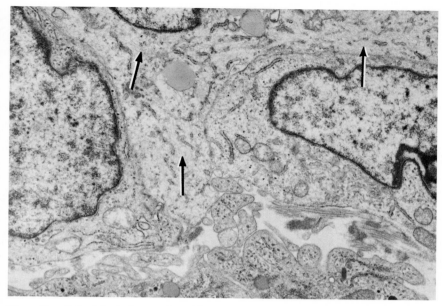

Figure 18.   Cells of the fetal mesenchymal hamartoma are of secondary mesenchyme; thus they do not produce basement membranes as do mesoblasts or more differentiated epithelial cells, although rudimentary attachment sites may be seen occasionally. The intercellular stroma contains loose bundles of collagen and aggregates of mucopolysaccharidelike material. The many microfilaments throughout the cytoplasm (straight arrows) are remarkable. (E.M. 8640.00×).

the only significant one has been the fibroblastic line. Light microscopic studies initially suggested a prominent smooth muscle component, but this has not been confirmed by electron microscopy.[66,67,70]

FMH has been virtually restricted to the neonatal period and has not been known to metastasize.[66,69] Tumors resembling it have, however, been discovered in older patients.[13,71,72] Whether all represent fetal hamartomas that may have matured or spontaneously ceased to grow is still unresolved. Since tumors have been known to change their biologic behavior with age,[73] one should be wary of renal connective tissue tumors beyond the newborn period. Furthermore, sarcomatous development has been reported in older patients with hamartomas.[47,48]

ORIGIN OF WILMS' TUMOR, THE VARIANTS, AND HAMARTOMATA AND THEIR RELATIONSHIPS

Wilms' tumor is a childhood tumor known to be associated with congenital malformation. To appreciate that an association of neoplasm and malformation is not unusual, one need only think of the connection between chromosomal aberration and leukemia in Down's syndrome,[74] or between hamartomatous syndromes such as von Recklinghausen's disease and malignant neural tumors.[47]

Many parallels exist between teratogenesis and carcinogenesis. Some drugs that have produced malformation while affecting immature cells can produce cancer when they affect mature cells. Other chemical agents administered during fetal life do not give rise to cancer until postnatal life. How can one explain the association of congenital malformation and neoplasm in early life? As one possible explanation, the concept has been advanced that cells responsive to differentiating or organizing influences can respond with teratogenesis, whereas cells, present simultaneously but beyond this stage, respond with neoplasia.[48,75]

No etiologic agent is known for Wilms' tumor, be it virus or carcinogen. Some light has, however, been shed on the pathogenesis of Wilms' tumor by comparison of data from familial Wilms' tumors, and from bilateral, unilateral, and unrelated Wilms' tumors, suggesting that the development of the tumor may be attributed to a two-mutational model.[53] This implies that two mutations are required in all cases, as was previously described for retinoblastoma; however, in about 38% one mutation has occurred in the germinal line of one parent and is inherited. In addition to the germinal mutant, a second mutation then results in the tumor. According to the model, about 37% of gene carriers do not develop tumor while 15% give rise to bilateral tumors. Approximately 62% of Wilms' tumors are nonhereditary, both mutations having occurred in somatic cells.[53]

The origin of cells affected by somatic mutations and producing Wilms' tumor is not definitely known. According to Cohnheim[17] and Wilms,[1] they should be cells of the nephrogenic mesoderm. This primary mesenchyme or mesoblast aggregates into an epithelium when forming the kidney anlage[76] and is called metanephric blastema. The ultrastructural appearance of these cells reveals definite epithelial characteristics and a remarkable similarity to the neoplastic cells. This finding led Ito and Johnson[35] to suggest that all neoplastic cells originating from the metanephric blastema differentiate into the epithelial components of Wilms' tumor. Since mesenchymal cells (in their least mature form called secondary mesenchyme) may be derived from mesodermal epithelia,[76] one might surmise that the connective tissue portion of Wilms' tumor is also derived from the metanephric blastema or the immature neoplastic epithelial cells. Secondary mesenchymal cells, however, never give rise to true epithelia. Striated muscle arises directly from epithelial cells, not from secondary mesenchyme.[77] One may, therefore, infer that Wilms' tumor and the fetal rhabdomyomatous nephroblastoma are tumors of mesoblast, whereas the fetal mesenchymal hamartoma is a tumor of secondary mesenchyme.

The normal period of induction of renal blastema ranges from 8 to 34 weeks gestation.[77] Thus it seems likely that germinal or somatic mutation would establish the nidus of Wilms' tumor during this period. Since in animal models of nephroblastoma the carcinogenic agent was applied beyond this period, the investigators presumed an origin from persistent nephronic elements.[40-42]

The origin and neoplastic potential of the multifocal epithelial hamartomata is still unresolved. Their incidence is certainly greater than that of Wilms' tumor; their marked fall in incidence after 4 months of age make it appear likely that most of these tumors will disappear spontaneously. On the other hand, 17% of these lesions were associated with Wilms' tumor,[50] especially bilateral Wilms' tumor. This fact has been interpreted as indirect evidence of a strong relationship between these hamartomata and Wilms' tumor.[53] The apparent maturation of the hamartomatous tissue in both the multifocal and the diffuse form in a case of nephroblastomatosis[61] indicates that these lesions must not be overtly neoplastic, that is, not a form of Wilms' tumor. The true incidence of multifocal hamartomata is not yet known. Their bilateral, disseminated distribution was believed to be consistent with an inherited alteration in renal cells, and their presence in bilateral and familial Wilms' tumor suggests a relationship to hereditary Wilms' tumor.[53]

SUMMARY

The histology of Wilms' tumor is reviewed with regard to its significance for prognosis. The histologic type has been shown to be an important factor influencing survival rate and cure rate. Electron microscopic techniques demonstrated that the least mature cells, the blastemal type, are epithelial in nature and are comparable to the cells of the metanephric anlage, thus indicating that Wilms' tumor is derived from mesoblast capable of forming both epithelial and mesenchymal cell lines.

The virtually monophasic mesenchymal variants of Wilms' tumor may contain neoplastic epithelial components, which suggests that they too are derived from mesoblast. The predominant differentiation into one connective tissue type, be it striped muscle, adipose tissue, or cartilage and bone, appears to have a beneficial influence on the prognosis of these tumors.

In contrast the hamartomas, both epithelial and mesenchymal, seem to be different. Fetal mesenchymal hamartoma, even in its least mature form, is composed of secondary mesenchymal cells or their derivatives, incapable of forming epithelia. This type of tumor is virtually restricted to the neonatal period. Epithelial hamartomas, although histologically similar to Wilms' tumor, probably mature or involute. The concomitant presence of the multifocal epithelial hamartoma with bilateral and familial Wilms' tumor suggests a relationship between them that has not yet been defined.

ACKNOWLEDGMENT

The technical and photographic assistance of Ms. K. Edwards and Ms. I. Nathan is gratefully acknowledged.

REFERENCES

1. Wilms, M.: *Die Mischgeschwülste*, Arthur Georgi, Leipzig, Germany, 1899, p. 1–90.

2. Bodian, M., and Rigby, C. C.: The pathology of nephroblastoma. In Riches, E., Ed.: *Tumors of the Kidney and Ureter*, vol. 5, Williams and Wilkins, Baltimore, 1964, pp. 219–234.

3. Kissane, J. M., and Smith, M. G.: *Pathology of Infancy and Childhood*, C. V. Mosby Company, St. Louis, 1967, pp. 583–586.

4. Anderson, W. A. D.: *Pathology*, C. V. Mosby Company, St. Louis, 1966, p. 651.

5. Anderson, W. A. D.: *Pathology*, C. V. Mosby Company, St. Louis, 1971, p. 822.

6. Robbins, S. L.: *Pathologic Basis of Disease*, ed. 2, W. B. Saunders Company, Philadelphia, 1974, pp. 1143–1144.

7. Ackerman, L. V., and Rosai, J.: *Surgical Pathology*, C. V. Mosby Company, St. Louis, 1974, pp. 658–660.

8. Fleming, I., and Pinkel, D.: Clinical staging of Wilms' tumor. *J. Pediatr.* **74**: 324–325, 1969.

9. Fleming, I. D., and Johnson, W. W.: Clinical and pathologic staging as a guide to the management of Wilms' tumor. *Cancer* **26**: 660–665, 1970.

10. Margolis, L. W., Smith, W. B., Wara, W., et al.: Wilms' tumor; an interdisciplinary treatment program with and without dactinomycin. *Cancer* **32**: 618–622, 1973.

11. Jereb, B., and Sandstedt, B.: Structure and size versus prognosis in nephroblastoma. *Cancer* **31**: 1473–1481, 1973.

12. Perez, C. A., Kaiman, H. A., Keith, J., et al.: Treatment of Wilms' tumor and factors affecting prognosis. *Cancer* **32**: 609–617, 1973.

13. Bolande, R. P., Brough, A. J., and Izant, R.: Congenital mesoblastic nephroma of infancy. *Pediatrics* **40**: 272–278, 1967.

14. Wigger, H. J.: Fetal hamartoma of kidney. *Am. J. Clin. Pathol.* **51**: 323–337, 1969.

15. Wigger, H. J.: Fetal rhabdomyoma or Wilms' tumor (abstr.) Pediatric Pathology Club Meeting, Toronto, Nov. 17, 1971.

16. Eberth, C. J.: Myoma sarcomatodes renum. *Virchows Arch.* **55**: 518–520, 1872.

17. Cohnheim, J.: Congenitales, quergestreiftes Muskelsarkom der Niere. *Virchows Arch. Pathol. Anat.* **65**: 64–69, 1875.

18. Hansen, J.: Quoted by Wilms(1). *Berl. Klin. Wochenschr.* p. 387, 1873.

19. Sturm, J.: Quoted by Wilms(1). *Arch. Heilk.* **35**: 232, 1875.

20. Birch-Hirschfeld, J.: Sarkomatöse Drüsengeschwülste der Niere im Kindesalter. *Beitr. z. Pathol. Anat. Allg. Pathol.* **24**: 532–539, 1896.

21. McCurdy, G. A.: Renal neoplasms in childhood. *J. Pathol. Bacteriol.* **39**: 623–633, 1934.

22. Culp, O. S., and Hartman, F. W.: Mesoblastic nephroma in adults; a clinico-pathologic study of Wilms' tumors and related renal neoplasma. *J. Urol.* **60**: 552–576, 1948.

23. Hedren, G.: Zur Kenntnis der Pathologie der Mischgeschwülste der Niere. *Beitr. z. Pathol. Anat. Allg. Pathol.* **40**: 1–107, 1907.

24. Nevinny, H.: Mesoblastische Mischgenschwüglste der Niere. Z. *Urol. Chir. Gynâk.* **20**: 295–400, 1926.

25. Herzog, H.: Nierengeschwülste mit quergestreifter Muskulatur. Z. *Krebsforsch.* **48**: 424–446, 1938.

26. Lieberthal, F.: Malignant tumors of the kidney in childhood. *Surg. Gynec. Obstet.* **11**: 77–88, 1931.

27. Stowens, D.: *Pediatric Pathology*, Williams and Wilkins, Baltimore, 1966, pp. 658–664.

28. Lattimer, J. K., Melicow, M. M., and Uson, A. C.: Nephroblastoma (Wilms' tumor); prognosis more favorable in infants under one year of age. *JAMA* **171**: 2163–2168, 1959.

29. Marsden, H. B., and Steward, J. K.: *Recent Results in Cancer Research*, (Vol. 13), Springer-Verlag, New York, 1968, p. 230.

30. Garcia, M., Douglas, C., and Schlosser, J. V.: Classification and prognosis of Wilms' tumor. *Radiology* **80**: 574–580, 1963.

31. Knutrud, O.: Nephroblastoma or Wilms' tumor, prognosis and treatment. *Acta Pathol. Microbiol. Scand.* (Suppl.) **51**: 146–150, 1961.

32. Contreras, F., Claver, M., and Picazo, M. L.: Criterios anatomopatologicos en la evolución del nefroblastome. *Rev. Clin. Esp.* **124**: 23–32, 1972.

33. Bannayan, G. A., Huvos, H. G., and D'Angio, G. J.: Effect of irradiation on the maturation of Wilms' tumor. *Cancer* **27**: 812–818, 1971.

37. Hajdu, S. I.: Exfoliative cytology of primary and metastatic Wilms' tumors. *Acta Cytol.* **15**: 339–342, 1971.

35. Ito, J., and Johnson, W. W.: Ultrastructure of Wilms' tumor. I. Epithelial Cell. *J. Natl. Cancer Inst.* **42**: 77–99, 1969.

36. Tannenbaum, M.: Ultrastructural pathology of human renal cell tumors. *Pathol. Ann.* **6**: 249–277, 1971.

37. Rousseau, M. F., and Nabarra, B.: Tumeurs embryonnaires du rein. *Virchows Arch. Pathol. Anat.* **363**: 149–162, 1974.

38. Balsaver, A. M., Gibley, C. W., and Tessmer, C. F.: Ultrastructural studies in Wilms' tumor. *Cancer* **22**: 417–427, 1968.

39. Trembley, M.: Ultrastructure of a Wilms' tumor and myogenesis. *J. Pathol.* **105**: 269–277, 1971.

40. Ishiguro, H., Beard, D., Sommer, J. R., et al.: Multiplicity of cell response to the BAI strain (myeloblastosis) and avian tumor virus. I. Nephroblastoma (Wilms' tumor); gross and microscopic pathology. *J. Natl. Cancer Inst.* **29**: 1–39, 1962.

41. Heine, U., de The, G., Ishiguro, H., et al.: Multiplicity of cell response to the BAI strain (myeloblastosis) and avian tumor virus, II. Nephroblastoma (Wilms' tumor); ultrastructure. *J. Natl. Cancer Inst.* **29**: 41–105, 1962.

42. Gusak, W.: Feinstruktur und Differenzierung experimenteller Wilmstumoren. *Verh. Dtsch. Ges. Pathol.* **52**: 410–415, 1968.

43. Tomashefsky, P., Furth, J., Lattimer, J. K., et al.: The Furth-Columbia rat Wilms' tumor. *J. Urol.* **108**: 348–354, 1972.

44. Ragab, A. H., Vietti, T. J., Christ, W., et al.: Bilateral Wilms' tumor; a review. *Cancer* **30**: 983–988, 1972.

45. Wigger, H. J., and Epstein, S. E.: Unpublished observations, 1974.

46. Weinberg, A. G.: Personal communication, 1974.

47. Jones, R., Jr., and Hart, D.: Discussion of multiple neurofibromatosis (von Recklinghausen's

disease); report of two cases having unusual surgical complications. *Ann. Surg.* **110**: 916–939, 1939.

48.   DiPaolo, J. A., and Kotin, P.: Teratogenesis-oncogenesis; a study of possible relationships. *Arch. Pathol.* **81**: 3–23, 1966.

49.   Shanklin, D. R., and Sotela-Avila, C.: In situ tumors in fetuses, newborns and young infants. *Biol. Neonat.* **14**: 286–316, 1969.

50.   Bove, K. E., Koffler, H., and McAdams, A. J.: Nodular renal blastema; definition and possible significance. *Cancer* **24**: 323–332, 1969.

51.   Liban, E., and Kosenitzky, I. L.: Metanephric hamartomas and nephroblastomatosis in siblings. *Cancer* **25**: 885–888, 1970.

52.   Hou, L. T., and Holman, R. L.: Bilateral nephroblastomatosis in a premature infant. *J. Pathol. Bacteriol.* **82**: 249–255, 1961.

53.   Knudson, A. G., and Strong, L. C.: Mutation and Cancer; a model for Wilms' tumor of the kidney. *J. Natl. Cancer Inst.* **48**: 313–324, 1972.

54.   Guin, G. H., Gilbert, E. F., and Jones, B.: Incidental neuroblastoma in infants. *Am. J. Clin. Pathol.* **51**: 126–136, 1969.

55.   Beckwith, J. B., and Perrin, E. V.: In situ neuroblastomas; a contribution to the natural history of neural crest tumors. *Am. J. Pathol.* **43**: 1089–1104, 1963.

56.   Bodian, M.: Neuroblastoma. *Pediatr. Clin. North Am.* **6**: 449–472, 1959.

57.   Pinkel, D., Dowd, J. E., and Bross, I. D. J.: Some epidemiologic features of malignant solid tumors of children in the Buffalo, New York area. *Cancer* **16**: 28–33, 1963.

58.   Lebreuil, G., Bérard-Badier, J., and Mariani, R.: La néphroblastomatose bilatérale; hyperplasie rénale par dysplasie polynéphronique. *Ann. Anat. Pathol. (Paris)* **15**:245–256, 1970.

59.   Vlachos, J., and Tsakraklides, V.: A case of renal dysplasia and relation to bilateral nephroblastomatosis. *J. Pathol. Bact.* **95**: 560–562, 1968.

60.   Perlman, M., Goldberg, G. M., Bar-Ziv, J., and Danovitch, G.: Renal hamartomas and nephroblastomatosis with fetal gigantism; a familial syndrome. *J. Pediatr.* **83**: 414–418, 1973.

61.   Mankad, V. N., Gray, G. F., and Miller, D. R.: Bilateral nephroblastomatosis and Klippel-Trenaunay Syndrome. *Cancer* **33**: 1462–1467, 1974.

62.   Fahr, T., and Lubarsch, O.: Die Nierengewäehse. In Henke, F., and Lubarsch, O. (Eds.): *Handbuch der speziellen pathologischen Anatomie and Histologie*, (vol. 6), Julius Springer, Berlin, 1925, p. 685.

63.   Potter, E. L.: *Pathology of the Fetus and Infant*, ed. 2, Year Book Medical Publishers, Chicago, 1961, p. 201.

64.   Zuckerman, I. C., Kershner, D., Laytner, B. D., and Hirschl, D.: Leiomyoma of the kidney. *Ann. Surg.* **126**: 220–228, 1947.

65.   Muto, K.: Renal sarcoma in a seven month fetus. *Gann* **34**: 77–214, 1940(abstr.); *JAMA* **116**: 786, 1941.

66.   Wigger, H. J.: Fetal mesenchymal hamartoma of kidney; a tumor of secondary mesenchyme. *Cancer*. In Press.

67.   Fu, Y. S., and Kay, S.: Congenital mesoblastic nephroma and its recurrence. *Arch. Pathol.* **96**: 66–70, 1973.

68.   Walker, D., and Richard, G. A.: Fetal hamartoma of the kidney: recurrence and death of patient. *J. Urol.* **110**: 352–353, 1973.

69.   Berdon, W. E., Wigger, H. J., and Baker, D. H.: Fetal renal hamartoma; a benign tumor to be distinguished from Wilms' tumor. *Am. J. Roentgenol.* **98**: 18–27, 1973.

70. Garcia-Bunuel, R., and Brandes, R.: Fetal hamartoma of kidney; case report with ultrastructural and cytochemical observation. *Johns Hopkins Med. J.* **127**: 213–221, 1970.

71. Early, R., Brown, B., and Terplan, K.: Fibroblastoma of renal parenchyma. *J. Urol.* **80**: 417–419, 1958.

72. Block, N. L., Grabstald, H. G., and Melamed, M. R.: Congenital mesoblastic nephroma (leiomyomatous hamartoma); first adult case. *J. Urol.* **110**: 380–383, 1973.

73. Bolande, R. P.: Benignity of neonatal tumors and concept of cancer repression in early life. *Am. J. Dis. Child* **122**: 12–14, 1971.

74. Gunz, F. W., and Fitzgerald, P. H.: Chromosomes and leukemia. *Blood* **23**: 394–400, 1964.

75. Miller, R. W., Fraumeni, J. F., Jr., and Manning, M. D.: Association of Wilms' tumor with aniridia, hemihypertrophy and other congenital malformations. *N. Engl. J. Med.* **270**: 922–927, 1964.

76. Trelstad, R. L., Hay, E. D., and Revel, J. P.: Cell contact during early morphogenesis in the chick. *Dev. Biol.* **16**: 78–106, 1967.

77. Potter, E. L.: Development of the human glomerulus. *Arch. Pathol.* **80**: 241–255, 1965.

CHAPTER EIGHT

Diagnostic Workup of the Child Suspected of Having Wilms' Tumor

D. G. YOUNG, M.D., M.B., B.S.

Department of Pediatric Surgery
Royal Hospital for Sick Children
Senior Lecturer
University of Glasgow
Yorkhill, Glasgow, Scotland

CONTENTS

I n 1814, in his introduction to a case presentation of probable Wilms' tumor in a 17-month-old infant, Rance wrote:

> However true it may be that some diseases baffle the skill of the medical practitioner, resisting all his curative and palliative attempts yet these disappointments ought never so to influence his mind as to damp his exertions, or restrain his endeavors in acquiring a more accurate knowledge of the malady under which his patient labours; for as diseases become the more difficult to remove, so should his researches become the more unwearied and assiduous; and if from the nature of the complaint his attempts at restoration or relief prove unavailing, he will generally find some recompense from the knowledge he has acquired in forming a more decisive diagnosis and correct prognosis.[1]

Establishing the diagnosis of Wilms' tumor in all patients when the tumor is limited to the kidney and the prognosis is good, remains a goal at which we aim but fall far short. There is little evidence that any significant advance has been made in this aspect in the past decade. Were this aim achieved, there would be little morbidity and mortality from Wilms' tumor. The best approach to successful treatment is early diagnosis and prompt treatment rather than the more complex therapy necessary for metastatic disease. In this latter group significant improvements in therapy have been achieved over the last 15 years.

As in many diseases, the prime factor in establishing an early diagnosis is an awareness of the possibility of encountering the disease by nurses and doctors attending infants and young children. Every routine examination of an infant or young child should include careful palpation of the abdomen for the presence of a mass. Careful abdominal palpation is an even more important part of the examination of a young patient who is ill, since the symptomatology of Wilms' tumor is usually nonspecific. Usually the presence of an abdominal mass is the first sign and is present in almost all patients with Wilms' tumor. Delay in diagnosis until there is a large, visible abdominal mass or until there are signs caused by metastasis, as in the child presenting with "bronchitis" or respiratory signs caused by pulmonary metastasis, results in the poorer chance of survival.

Discussion of the diagnostic workup of the child with Wilms' tumor will be considered under three headings: (1) clinical presentation, (2) investigations, and (3) staging the disease. Each of these are interrelated and, although separation is artificial, it is useful in considering this topic.

CLINICAL PRESENTATION

Although Wilms' tumor is a relatively common cause of death in childhood, it is not a common disease and the incidence is about 1:10,000 births,[2] or 2:1,000,000 where the age distribution is that of the developed nations of the Western world.

Thus doctors or nurses whose practices are limited to children will encounter very few cases of Wilms' tumor during their professional career unless they work specifically in cancer therapy.

Adding to the difficulties of early diagnosis of Wilms' tumor is the young age group in which the disease occurs. Eighty percent of patients are diagnosed before school age (5 years), and the second year of life is the age of peak incidence.[3] Because of this an adequate history of symptomatology is unobtainable. Although abdominal pain, fever, and/or vomiting occur in approximately half the patients,[4] these are nonspecific signs, as are lethargy, irritability, and altered bowel habit. Hematuria suggests of a urinary tract neoplasm, but Aron[4] found it in 10% of patients, and in Glasgow it was present in only 5%. In adults, hematuria is an important sign of neoplasia in the urinary tract. In pediatrics, most patients presenting with hematuria have benign conditions. There is no contraindication to an early intravenous pyelogram in young patients and it is necessary for early diagnosis of Wilms' tumor.

An abdominal mass is almost always palpable,[3,-5] and may be noted on examination or may have been detected earlier by the child's parents. This mass is usually firm and often large, and the most immediate condition from which it must be differentiated is neuroblastoma. When the patient is examined from behind, Wilms' tumor fills up the renal angle; this is not a feature in the patient with neuroblastoma. Palpation, which should be minimal in case of rupturing of disseminating tumor, reveals a firm, usually smooth mass which enlarges up or down in the paravertebral gutter. Although Wilms' tumor does not usually cross the midline, there are exceptions. When the tumor is large it spreads across the midline, or when the tumor arises in a horseshoe kidney or an ectopic kidney it may cross the midline, and in bilateral Wilms' tumor masses may appear to be continuous across the midline.

A group of infants and children who should be considered at risk of developing Wilms' tumor are those in whom conditions known to occur in association with this malignancy are present. The best known of these are aniridia, hemihypertrophy, and some genitourinary tract malformations.[6,7] Also, the increased frequency of Wilms' tumor in twin sibs and recent reports of familial cases[8] should make one particularly aware of such groups of patients, to insure early detection of possible disease.

INVESTIGATIONS

After the routine clinical examination of a patient in whom an abdominal tumor has been found, immediate investigation of the nature of this mass should be undertaken. With suspected Wilms' tumor, the investigations are mainly of the urine and radiological examination.

Urine

Apart from routine examination of the urine, concentrating the cellular deposit and examining it for the presence of malignant cells has been carried out on many patients. These cytologic studies have not been very useful,[9] since tumor cells have been found in the urine only where Wilms' tumor has infiltrated into the collecting system. The examination is very time-consuming and gives too few positive results to be of value. A 6- or 24-hour collection of urine is also made because there is clinical difficulty in separating Wilms' tumor from neuroblastoma. The level of the catecholamine excretion products in the urine is normal in Wilms' tumor but elevated in neuroblastoma.

Radiology

The mainspring of diagnosis is radiologic investigation—initially an intravenous pyelogram (IVP) and a chest x-ray (see Chapter 2). Although the IVP shows distortion of the normal caliceal pattern, there is no single characteristic pattern since the distortion varies with the site of origin of the tumor, the size of the tumor at investigation, and possible spread of the tumor into the renal vein. Where the IVP proves inadequate, an infusion pyelogram usually gives better definition. Chest x-ray is important at the outset to determine if there is any evidence of pulmonary secondaries, since this affects staging and treatment. Unfortunately pulmonary secondaries, which are only a few millimeters or less in diameter, are not detectable on x-ray examination. This is one source of potential error in staging which has not been overcome. Skeletal survey, especially with reference to the skull, dorsal lumbar sacral spine, and long bones, is recommended by some clinicians in search of bony lesions but is rarely, if ever, positive if chest xray is negative.

Many further radiologic investigations may be undertaken and are done as a routine in some clinics. Most of these technically impressive procedures are unnecessary. They prolong diagnosis, which usually is established on clinical and pyelography findings, and delay the institution of effective treatment. These include retrograde pyelography, which probably had a place before good excretory pyelograms could be obtained but seldom contributes anything further to diagnosis or treatment planning. Aortography and selective renal arteriography[10] are marked advances in further radiologic investigation and are frequently used in some centers. Although it provides some further information, this investigation is seldom indicated since it does not alter the course of management in unilateral cases. If arteriography has a place, it is in the patient with bilateral tumors. The second objection to arteriography is that it is not always correct because the tumor blush which should be seen may occasionally be absent and thus give the misleading impression of a benign cyst.

A less frequently performed procedure that provides information in an occasional patient is venography.[11] With venography the surgeon can be forewarned of extension of tumor into the vena cava, and he will therefore be prepared to remove it when performing the nephrectomy. However, naked eye inspection at laparotomy will reveal this extension of tumor. Lymphangiography in the young age group is technically difficult and, since paraaortic glands are going to be excised and examined histologically for evidence of infiltration, there is little place for this examination. Renal scanning can provide further evidence of Wilms' tumor and of the remaining renal tissue. Renograms are not of value because they show nonspecific changes which do not differentiate Wilms' tumor from other lesions.

A more recent development which helps to differentiate Wilms' tumor from other renal masses is ultrasonic scanning. In experienced hands this examination is simple, noninvasive, and causes minimal upset to the patient. It may be done at the same time as the IVP and shows the large tumor mass with irregular echoes compared with the normal renal outline of the nonaffected kidney, with echoes delineating the normal pelvis (Figure 1). Figure 2 shows a longitudinal scan of a child with a very large Wilms' tumor occupying the left side of the abdomen; the transverse scan (Figure 1) shows that the tumor extends across the midline in front of the right renal pelvis. Figure 3 shows a transverse prone view of the ultrasound examination of the same child outlining the normal kidney (right), with the echoes indicating the pelvis and calices.

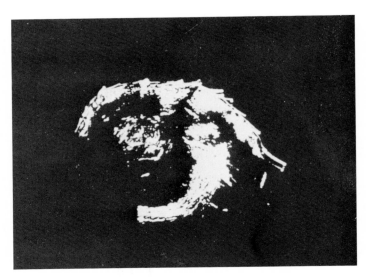

Figure 1.   Ultrasound examination. Transverse scan showing large tumor on the left and normal renal outline on the right. Tumor is crossing midline and encroaching on right kidney.

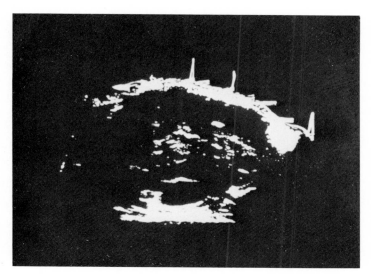

Figure 2. Longitudinal ultrasonic scan. Right-hand marker is at pubic level and central one at umbilical level. Examination shows large tumor mass extending down and almost reaching the pubis.

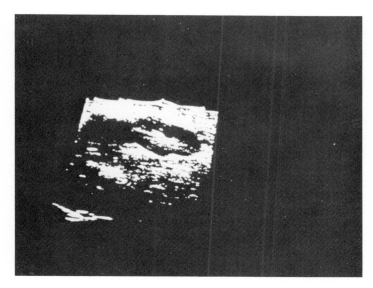

Figure 3. Prone ultrasonic scan showing the normal-sized right kidney.

Other investigations, such as bone marrow examination, rarely show tumor cells in patients with Wilms' tumor.[12] Blood examination has shown raised levels of acid mucopolysaccharides occasionally,[13] but this has not been useful in detecting recurrence or regression of tumor. Currently the α-fetoprotein level, which has been found elevated in a number of different conditions, is being investigated as a possible indicator of recurrence of tumor. Although elevated levels have been found in recurrence of other embryonic tumors its value in Wilms' tumor is not yet defined. Blood chemistries that include BUN, SGOT, and perhaps alkaline phosphatase, should be done to serve as a baseline for future comparison.

CLASSIFYING THE DISEASE

In the various attempts made to subdivide patients with Wilms' tumor into comparable groups three main factors have been used: age, histologic appearance, and spread of tumor.

Age appeared to be a major factor in defining prognosis since younger patients, particularly those under 1 year of age, have a better prognosis. It now seems clear that two factors contributed to this. First, in this group there were a number of patients with "congenital Wilms' tumor," a disease with a different behavior and prognosis (see Chapter 9). The second and more important factor became apparent on closer analysis of these patients: at surgery there was a higher proportion of patients with tumor localized in the kidney.[14]

Staging

An attempt was also made to classify these patients by the histologic type of the tumor. This method was not of much value in determining the prognosis,[15] and has not been useful in determining the appropriate therapeutic approach. Similarly, although staging based on the gross volume of the tumor was not generally accepted,[16] the current classification system has gradually evolved from this method.

The current practice of classifying patients with Wilms' tumor has become worldwide, and it is probable that in the near future universal acceptance of classification along the lines shown in Table 1 will be standard.

This type of staging proved of value in American, British, and European trials currently in progress. It allows more meaningful comparison of results and may help in time to elucidate the best chemotherapeutic approach or combination therapy for children with tumor which has spread beyond the renal capsule. To achieve correct staging of patients it is, therefore, essential that adequate tissue be submitted to the pathologist for histologic examination. It is no longer satisfactory for the surgeon to look at paraaortic glands and guess whether they are involved or

Table 1.   Criteria for Clinical Staging of Wilms' Tumors

Stage I.	A well-encapsulated tumor which is entirely removed at operation. Spillage of the tumor does not take place during operation and there is no involvement of the para-aortic nodes on biopsy.
Stage II.	Extension of the tumor beyond the renal capsule either by: (a) local infiltration, or (b) extension along the renal vein, or (c) involvement of the para-aortic glands, but the surgeon believes total removal of macroscopic disease was possible.
Stage III.	Extension of the tumor beyond the renal capsule and (a) spillage of tumor at operation, or (b) when tumor is felt to have been left at operation, or (c) there are peritoneal metastases.
Stage IV.	Spread to lung, liver, bone, or brain is found at diagnosis.
Stage V.	Bilateral disease.

are the site of nonspecific reactive hyperplasia. Excision and histologic examination are essential for correct staging. Unfortunately, the problem already referred to of the relatively late time at which pulmonary secondaries become radiologically visible remains unanswered. At present, since this does not lend itself to more precise definition for correct staging, this error must be accepted.

Lest this discussion leave the reader with the impression that there is never any problem in diagnosing Wilms' tumor, it must be stressed that this is not so. In 1828, describing a patient with probable Wilms' tumor, Gairdner commented: "Upwards of 70 years ago indeed, Morgagni declared that he, as well as Valsalva, found the diagnosis of the diseases of the kidneys and urinary organs to be uncertain and fallacious."[17] Although medicine may have advanced, the end of the road has not been reached in diagnosis, as is indicated by reports from the combined trials in which erroneous preoperative diagnosis continues to occur. Currently, adequate clinical awareness and experience and good radiologic investigation minimize the problems encountered and, with the occasional addition of ultrasonography, accurate diagnosis should be achieved. Classification is now generally accepted along the lines indicated.

SUMMARY

Since early diagnosis of Wilms' tumor is vital, clinical awareness is of prime importance. Presenting symptoms are usually nonspecific. The most common sign is an abdominal mass usually confined to one side of the abdomen with fullness in that loin. Abdominal palpation should be a routine part of all examinations of infants and children. The most important examination is the intravenous pyelogram, which should be performed urgently. In patients in whom doubt about the diagnosis remains after this examination, ultrasound examination of the abdomen will be useful. Venography aids in delineating growth of the tumor along the renal vein into the vena cava. Aortography and selective renal arteriography are additional procedures that may be performed. Staging depends on chest x-ray and laparotomy findings and subsequent histologic examination of the excised tumor and glands.

ACKNOWLEDGMENT

The ultrasonograms were supplied by Dr. Margaret McNair of the Radiology Department, Royal Hospital for Sick Children, Glasgow.

REFERENCES

1. Rance, T. F.: A case of fungus haematodes in the kidney. *Med. Phys. J.* **32**:19, 1814.
2. Cochran, W., and Frogatt, P.: Bilateral nephroblastoma in two sisters. *J. Urol.* **97**:216–220, 1967.
3. Young, D. G., and Williams, D. I.: Malignant renal tumours of infancy and childhood. *Br. J. Hosp. Med.* **2**:741–752, 1969.
4. Aron, B. S.: Wilms' tumor; a clinical study of 81 patients. *Cancer* **33**:637–646, 1974.
5. Milligan, G. F., and Young, D. G.: Nephroblastoma in childhood. *Scot. Med. J.* **16**:317–321, 1971.
6. Miller, R. W., Fraumeni, J. F., and Manning, M. D.: Association of Wilms' tumour with aniridia, hemihypertrophy and other congenital malformations. *N. Engl. J. Med.* **270**:922–927, 1964.
7. DiGeorge, A. M., and Harley, R. D.: The association of aniridia, Wilms' tumour and genital abnormalities. *Arch. Ophthalmol.* **75**:796–798, 1966.
8. Brown, W. T., Puranik, S. R., Altman, D. H., and Hardin, H. C., Jr.: Wilms' tumour in three successive generations. *Surgery* **72**:(5):756–761, 1972.
9. Helson, L., and Hajdu, S. I.: The cytology of urine of pediatric cancer patients. *J. Urol.* **108**:660–662, 1972.
10. Farrah, J., and Lofstrom, J. E.: Angiography of Wilms' tumour. *Radiology* **90**:775–777, 1968.
11. Tucker, A. S.: The roentgen diagnosis of abdominal masses in children. *Am. J. Roentgenol.* **95**:76–90, 1965.
12. O'Neill, P., and Pinkel, D.: Wilms' tumour in bone marrow aspirate. *J. Pediatr.* **72**:396–398, 1968.
13. Morse, B. S., and Nussbaum, M.: Detection of hyaluronic acid in the serum and urine of a patient with nephroblastoma. *Am. J. Med.* **42**:996–1002, 1967.
14. Fleming, I. D., and Johnston, W. W.: Clinical and pathologic staging as a guide in the management of Wilms' tumour. *Cancer* **26**:660–665, 1970.
15. Bodian, M., and Rigby, C. C.: The pathology of nephroblastoma. In Riches, E., Ed.: *Tumours of the kidney and ureter*, E. and S. Livingstone, London, 1964, p. 219.
16. Garcia, M., Douglass, C., and Schlosser, J. V.: Classification and prognosis in Wilms' tumour. *Radiology* **80**:574–580, 1963.
17. Gairdner, E.: Case of fungus haematodes in the kidneys. *Edinb. Med. Surg. J.* **29**:312, 1828.

CHAPTER NINE

Bilateral Wilms' Tumor: Pathogenesis, Diagnosis, and Treatment

HARRY S. DAVID, M.D.

Chief Resident (Urology)
St. Luke's Hospital Center
Visiting Clinical Fellow (Urology)
College of Physicians and Surgeons
Columbia University
and
Department of Urology
St. Luke's Hospital Center
New York, New York

CONTENTS

There are many opinions about the treatment and management of bilateral Wilms' tumor. There is even conflicting evidence about the incidence of bilateral Wilms' tumor and whether they represent two separate primary tumors or metastasis from the first kidney to the second. In this chapter a case of bilateral Wilms' tumor will be described,[1] and followed by a discussion on the pathogenesis, treatment, and management of this clinical entity as they have evolved over the past several decades.

REPORT OF A CASE

A 17-month-old boy was admitted to St. Luke's Hospital Center in January, 1971, for evaluation of an enlarged abdomen and extreme thirst. The infant was the product of a full-term pregnancy and weighed 8 lb at birth. The mother stated that the infant had always had a large abdomen but noted further enlargement a few weeks prior to admission. There was no past history of urinary tract infection.

Physical examination revealed an irritable, emaciated, chronically ill-looking infant. His pulse rate was 164/min, temperature 99.8°F and weight was 19 lb 13 oz. Positive physical findings were confined to the abdomen, which revealed bilateral masses extending from 2 to 3 cm below the costal margins to the pelvis. There was no apparent tenderness. The complete blood count, urinalysis, and determination of serum electrolytes were within normal limits. Urine culture showed no growth, and the blood urea nitrogen (BUN) was 24 mg%. An intravenous pyelogram (IVP) showed bilateral severe hydronephrosis with marked loss of renal parenchyma, bilaterally (Figure 1). The picture suggested bilateral ureteropelvic obstruction with less obstruction in the right excretory system. For this reason the right kidney was initially explored transabdominally to correct the ureteral obstruction. At operation, bilateral renal tumors were noted. The left kidney was found to be totally involved with tumor. Tumor also appeared to involve the lower two-thirds of the right kidney with invasion of the hilum. Biopsy of both kidneys revealed Wilms' tumor.

Since the National Wilms' Tumor Study Group has no official protocol for Stage V (bilateral Wilms' tumor), the decision was made to treat our patient as if he were Stage IV. He was placed on a regimen of chemotherapy and radiotherapy. Accordingly, the patient received 1430 rads of radiotherapy to the entire abdomen and 300 rads to the left kidney (the most affected). Actinomycin D, at a dose of 0.015 mg/kg/day for 5 days, was started within 48 hr of surgery and vincristine, 1.5mg/m^2, was given on day 7, then weekly for 8 weeks. According to protocol, chemotherapy consisting of 5 daily courses of actinomycin D together with 2 doses of vincristine, 1 each on the first and fifth days of administration of actinomycin D, were to be repeated at 6 weeks and at 3, 6, 9, 12, and 15 months. The infant received only one repeated course of chemotherapy at 6 weeks. Two days after

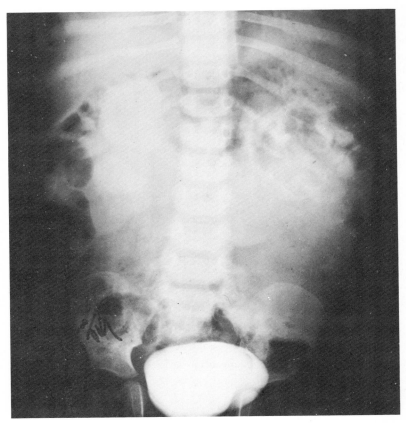

Figure 1.   Preoperative intravenous pyelogram, showing bilateral hydronephrosis (Courtesy of *Urology*.[1])

completion of the course nausea, vomiting, and fever developed. The child was hospitalized for 5 days and responded well to intravenous fluids. The infant's mother refused further chemotherapy until October, 1972, 21 months postdiagnosis. The patient's general health at this time was good and, because of the improved prognosis for patients with Wilms' tumor who receive long-term intermittent chemotherapy, the chemotherapy schedule was restarted as though we were at the 3-month postoperative stage.

The patient tolerated chemotherapy so well that the possibility of renal transplant was considered. Since our hospital was not equipped to handle pediatric hemodialysis, he was transferred to The New York Hospital-Cornell Medical Center for further management. In January, 1973, he underwent a metastatic workup which included liver, spleen, and bone scans. All findings were normal.

The chest x-ray and bone marrow examination were also normal. The BUN was 29 mg% and serum creatinine was 0.8 mg% at this time. Chemotherapy was continued. However, an IVP performed on this admission revealed nonvisualization of the left kidney with marked increase in calcification at that site (Figure 2). The child's parents consented to a reexploration of his kidneys but stipulated that only one kidney should be removed at this time, since they could not accept

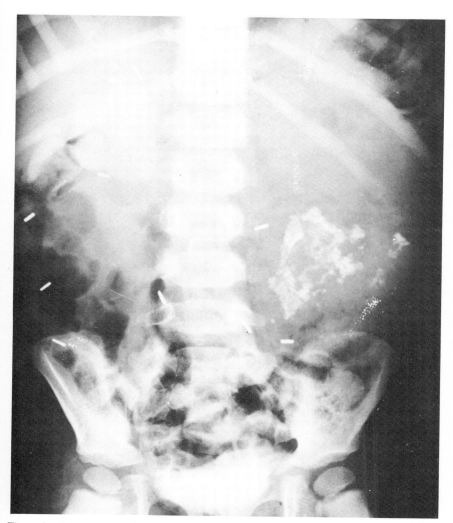

Figure 2. Intravenous pyelogram taken prior to reexploration of both kidneys. (Courtesy of Urology.[1])

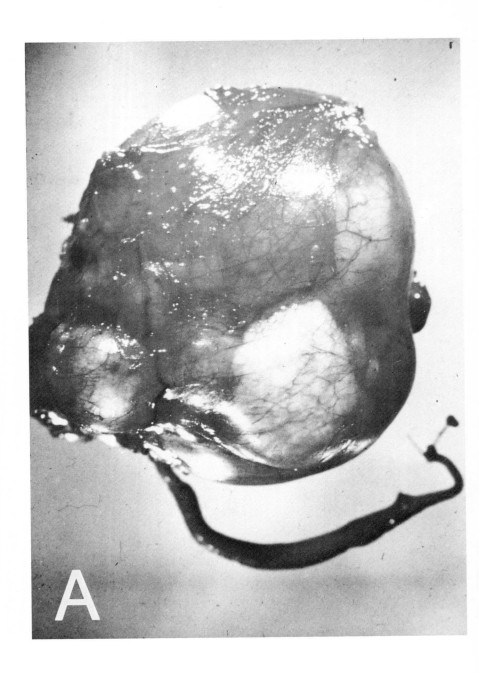

A

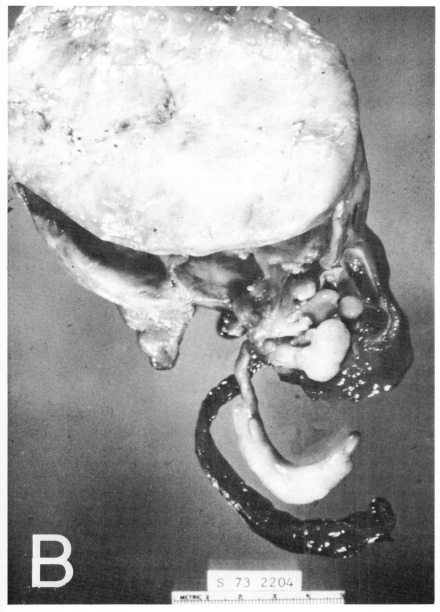

Figure 3. Gross specimen of left kidney. *(A)* Intact surgical specimen. *(B)* Section showing tumor extending downward within the ureter. (Courtesy of Urology.[1])

chronic hemodialysis and renal transplantation. In March, a left radical nephrectomy was performed through a chevron incision. Tumor was found to extend down the proximal one-third of the left ureter (Figure 3). Microscopic examination of the tumor revealed posttherapy fibrotic changes but, in addition, nests of malignant cells were found throughout the specimen. The right kidney was found to be totally involved with tumor at this time. Later that year, the parents consented to renal transplantation; and on April 24, 1973, the child underwent a right nephrectomy and allotransplantation. The child rejected this first kidney transplant and underwent a second transplant on May 4, 1973. On October 5, 5 months following the second transplant, the patient died. Death was due to pneumonia, probably a complication of the immunosuppressive therapy.

DISCUSSION

> However true it may be that some diseases baffle the skill of the medical practitioner, resisting all his curative and palliative attempts, yet these disappointments ought never so to influence his mind as to damp his exertions, or restrain his endeavours in acquiring a more accurate knowledge of the malady under which his patient labors, for as diseases become more difficult to remove, so should his researches become the more unwearied and assiduous. . . .[2]

This is a quote from a paper by Rance, who in 1814 reported the first renal tumor in a child, a case of bilateral Wilms' tumor. These words adequately express the feelings of frustration and despair one often experiences when dealing with malignancy during childhood. When these are renal and there is bilateral involvement, these feelings soon turn to hopelessness and gloom. Careful review of the advances in treatment and management of bilateral Wilms' tumor may lessen the feelings of despair associated with the diagnosis of this clinical entity.

More than 120 cases of bilateral Wilm's tumor are listed in the literature. (Table 1). The reported incidence of bilateral disease ranges from 1.4%[3] to as high as 11.6%[4] of all Wilms' tumors. Creevey and Reiser[5] reported 28 cases of bilateral involvement of 1170 cases of Wilms' tumor, giving an incidence of 2.3%. Scott[6] reported 33 cases out of 906 cases of Wilms' tumor studied by his group, or an incidence of 3.6%. Gross and Neuhauser[7] reported an incidence of 4.1%, while Ragab[4] reported 5 of bilateral involvement out of 43 cases of Wilms' tumor, an incidence of 11.6%. The overall incidence in 3609 cases is 3.3%.

The diagnosis is most commonly suspected by the parent or physician when a large hard mass is palpated, or when abdominal distention is noted. Pain is the next most common symptom and is the chief complaint in 30% of cases. Unlike renal tumors in adults, urinary complaints are rare. Hematuria is present in only 10% of cases, and carries with it an extremely poor prognosis.[3]

Physical examination reveals a hard mass in either upper quadrant or bilaterally

Table 1. Reported Incidence of Bilateral Wilms' Tumor

Author	Number of Wilms' Tumors	Number of Bilateral Tumors	Percent of Bilateral Tumors
Creevy and Reiser[5]	1170	28	2.3
Scott[6]	906	33	3.6
Abeshouse[3]	856	12	1.4
Jagasia et al.[8]	116	12	10.3
Bishop and Hope[14]	78	6	8.3
Gross and Neuhauser[7]	96	4	4.1
Rickham[15]	25	2	8.0
Walker[19]	141	10	7.0
Ragab et al.[4]	43	5	11.6
Martin and Kloecher[17]	39	3	7.7
Gross (cited by Martin)[17]	139	6	4.3
Total	3609	121	3.3

palpable masses. Fever may be present, especially when there is tissue necrosis. Blood pressure may be elevated. An IVP may reveal mechanical distortion of the renal pelvis, obstruction of the ureters with hydronephrosis, or one or both kidneys may not visualize. Retrograde pyelography can be employed if the IVP is unsatisfactory. Sonography and arteriography may prove useful in obtaining the proper diagnosis.

Pathogenesis

Whether bilateral Wilms' tumor represents separate primary growths or metastasis from one kidney to the other is not definitely known. There is evidence which supports both theories. After reviewing the literature, Scott[6] suggested that the majority of reported cases represented metastatic spread from one kidney to the other. Jagasia et al.[8] reviewed the evidence supporting the theory of *separate primaries* which includes:

1. At operation or at autopsy, no evidence of direct tumor extension across the midline is noted.
2. Simultaneous involvement of both kidneys was found in 65% of cases[9] with no evidence of metastases to other sites.
3. Clumps of primitive blastoma cells made up most of the tumors in both kidneys, this being an indication of abnormal growth in situ.[10]
4. There is no evidence of other metastases found at the time of discovery of tumor in the second kidney.

5. Metastatic lesions have been reported in other organs, such as lung or liver, but at autopsy no tumor is found in the other kidney.
6. Bilateral Wilms' tumor was found in a premature infant of 32 weeks' gestation by Hou and Holman,[11] and a similar finding in a 6½-month fetus was reported by Barrett and McCague.[12] These findings strongly suggest separate primary tumors because both kidneys showed uniform involvement at the same stages of development.

Jagasia cites the following as evidence supporting the *metastatic origin* of bilateral Wilms' tumor.

1. Multiple lesions are occasionally found in the remaining kidney.[8]
2. Bloodborne metastases are frequently seen in patients with Wilms' tumor.
3. Higher incidence of bilateral involvement is found in patients who died of advanced malignant disease where no treatment of the primary tumors was attempted. Scott quotes incidence figures which to him suggest that, if a tumor is left alone and allowed to progress to a fatal termination, it may in time metastasize to the opposite side.[6]

Thus it appears that there is more evidence suggesting the occurrence of separate primaries. In the case presented above, there was simultaneous Wilms' tumor with no evidence of metastases at surgery. Ritter and Scott[13] reported a delayed appearance of tumor in the opposite kidney as late as 10 years after an apparently successful nephrectomy. Since there were no other metastases elsewhere in the body, this case supports the argument for separate primary tumors.

Treatment

In children with Wilms' tumor, the presence of bilateral tumors should always be suspected. Special attention should be paid to the opposite kidney during the preoperative x-ray studies and at surgery. A wide transperitoneal incision (a chevron incision does very well) permits the surgeon to inspect and also to palpate the opposite kidney. If surgical exploration reveals only unilateral involvement, a cure cannot be claimed unless the child is followed closely with abdominal examinations and repeated IVPs. Cases have been reported of involvement of the opposite kidney from as early as 6 months[8] to as late as 10 years postoperatively.[13] Repeat IVPs should be done every 6 months for at least 4 to 6 years as suggested by DeLorimier, et al.[9] or perhaps until the child is at least 6 years old and is thus at an age where the incidence of Wilms' tumor is lower.[14]

There are several cases of cure of bilateral Wilms' tumor reported in the literature. Gross and Neuhauser[7] cited a case reported by Ladd in which the child was still alive 15 years after nephrectomy on one side and radiation therapy to the other. Scott[6] reported a 6-month survival for a child treated in a similar manner. Rickham[15] described a child who was alive and well 34 months after nephrectomy on one side and partial nephrectomy on the other. Flannery[16] reported a 5-year survival in a child in whom nephrectomy was performed on one side at age 14 months and a separate tumor was then removed from the other kidney 29 months later. Ragab et al.[4] reviewed 70 reported cases of bilateral Wilms' tumor and identified 28 cases that were considered cured, a survival rate of 40%. The authors admit that this is probably a falsely high survival rate because physicians are more apt to document their successes than their failures.

The above experience is presented to support the idea that bilateral Wilms' tumor does not necessarily carry a fatal prognosis. In the past, the treatment of bilateral Wilms' tumor has been limited to radiation therapy alone, a combination of radiation therapy and chemotherapy, a partial resection of both kidneys, or partial nephrectomy on one side and total nephrectomy on the other side with or without pre- and postoperative radiation. Martin and Kloecher[17] advocate bilateral heminephrectomy or partial nephrectomy on one side and total nephrectomy on the other at initial laparotomy, followed with a combination of x-ray therapy and chemotherapy. Bishop and Hope[14] suggest an approach involving three operative procedures: (1) bilateral kidney biopsies to confirm the diagnosis and to evaluate the extent of the tumors, (2) both kidneys are treated with radiation therapy and chemotherapy, giving no more than 800 rads of radiation therapy to the less involved kidney, and (3) wait 1 to 3 months and then reexplore the less involved kidney in the hope of doing a heminephrectomy. Finally, when the success of the heminephrectomy is certain, the contralateral more involved kidney can be completely removed. The effects of radiation therapy to the kidney have been studied by Vaeth;[18] he found no evidence of radiation nephritis with doses of radiation therapy varying from 1000 to 1500 rads.

A more vigorous approach to treatment has been advocated by DeLorimier et al.[9] They suggest bilateral nephrectomy and allotransplantation in cases in which the tumors are not radiosensitive, or in which both kidneys are diffusely involved, with tumor invading the hilar vessels making resection impossible. In 1968, DeLorimier et al.[9] were the first to report a case of simultaneous bilateral nephrectomy and renal allotransplantation in a small child with bilateral Wilms' tumor. In 1971, this group reported on 8 consecutive cases of bilateral Wilms' tumor they had treated. Of the 8 patients, 5 eventually underwent bilateral nephrectomy and renal transplantation. They reported 2 survivors and accounted for the 3 deaths as follows: 1 child died of distant metastasis, since liver metastasis was present at the time of transplant; 1 patient died of an intestinal fistula and sepsis that appeared to be related to multiple courses of radiation therapy and chemotherapy; and 1 child died of disseminated varicella infection, probably a complication of immunosuppressive therapy. They concluded that with more aggressive treatment of bilateral Wilms' tumor, one should be able to obtain survival rates equivalent to that of unilateral Wilms' tumor. They suggest that bilateral nephrectomy, hemodialysis, and allotransplantation should be performed as soon as radiation and chemotherapy have been shown to fail in controlling the tumor.

SUMMARY

A review of the literature reveals more than 120 cases of bilateral Wilms' tumor. The reported incidence of this clinical entity ranges from 1.4 to 11.6%. Two opposing theories have been proposed to explain the pathogenesis of bilateral Wilms' tumor, with the weight of evidence in favor of the occurrence of separate primaries. A great deal of progress has been made in therapy with improved techniques of chemotherapy and radiotherapy. With the advent of hemodialysis and allotransplantation, there appears to be hope for the cases where the tumors are neither resectable nor radiosensitive.

The management of bilateral Wilms' tumor should include:

1. Biopsy of both tumors.
2. Shrinkage or arrest of tumor growth by chemotherapy and radiation therapy as outlined by the protocol of the National Wilms' Tumor Study Group.
3. Heminephrectomy of the least involved side and removal of the more involved kidney.
4. In cases where the tumors are not radiosensitive, in cases in which both kidneys are diffusely involved with tumor, or in cases in which the tumors invade the hilar vessels making resection impossible, bilateral nephrectomy, hemodialysis, and renal transplantation is the treatment of choice.

REFERENCES

1. David, H. S., and Lavengood, R. W.: Bilateral Wilms' tumor treatment, management, and review of the literature. *Urology* **3**: 71, 1974.
2. Rance, T. E.: Cited by Rickham, P. P.[15] *Med. Phys. J.* **32**: 19, 1814.
3. Abeshouse, B. S.: The management of Wilms' tumor as determined by national survey and review of the literature. *J. Urol.* **77**: 792, 1957.
4. Ragab, A. H., Vietti, T. J., Crist, W., et al.: Bilateral Wilms' tumor; a review. *Cancer* **30**: 983, 1972.
5. Creevy, C. D., and Reiser, M. P.: Wilms' tumor. *Bull. Univ. Minn. Hosp. Minn. Med. Found.* **22**: 292, 1951.
6. Scott, L. S.: Bilateral Wilms' tumor. *Br. J. Surg.* **42**: 513, 1955.
7. Gross, R. E., and Neuhauser, E. B. D.: Treatment of mixed tumors of the kidney in childhood. *Pediatrics* **6**: 843, 1950.
8. Jagasia, K. H., Thurman, W. G., Pickett, E., and Grabstald, H.: Bilateral Wilms' tumor in children. *J. Pediatr.* **65**: 371, 1964.

9. DeLorimier, A. A., Belzer, F., Kountz, S., and Kushner, J.: Simultaneous bilateral nephrectomy and renal allotransplantation for bilateral Wilms' tumor. *Surgery* **64**: 850, 1968.

10. Bodian, M., and White, L. R.: (cited by Jagasia). Personal communication to Rickham, P. P., quoted in *Br. J. Surg.* **44**: 492, 1957.

11. Hou, L. T., and Holman, R. L.: Bilateral nephroblastoma in a premature infant. *J. Pathol. Bacteriol.* **82**: 249, 1961.

12. Barrett, W. A., and McCague, E. J.: Histopathology in prognosis of kidney tumors. *J. Urol.* **71**: 684, 1954.

13. Ritter, J. A., and Scott, E. S.: Embryoma of contralateral kidney ten years following nephrectomy for Wilms' tumor. *J. Pediatr.* **34**: 753, 1949.

14. Bishop, H. C., and Hope, J. W.: Bilateral Wilms' tumor. *J. Pediatr. Surg.* **1**: 476, 1966.

15. Rickham, P. P.: Bilateral Wilms' tumor. *Br. J. Surg.* **44**: 492, 1957.

16. Flannery, J. L.: Survival after nephrectomy and partial nephrectomy for bilateral Wilms' tumor. *U.S. Armed Forces Med. J.* **9**: 561, 1958.

17. Martin, L. W., and Kloecher, R. T.: Bilateral nephroblastoma. *Pediatrics* **28**: 101, 1961.

18. Vaeth, J. M.: The remaining kidney in irradiated survivors of Wilms' tumor. *Am. J. Roentgenol.* **92**: 148, 1964.

19. Walker, G.: Sarcoma of kidney in children; a critical review of the pathology, symptomatology, prognosis and operative treatment as seen in 145 cases. *Ann. Surg.* **26**: 529, 1897.

CHAPTER TEN

Congenital Wilms' Tumor

JOSEPH GIANGIACOMO, M.D.

Assistant Professor of Pediatrics
Pediatric Nephrology
St. Louis University School of Medicine
Cardinal Glennon Memorial Hospital for Children
St. Louis, Missouri

JOHN M. KISSANE, M.D.

Professor of Pathology
Washington University School of Medicine
Associate Pathologist
Barnes and Affiliated Hospitals and
St. Louis Children's Hospital
St. Louis, Missouri

CONTENTS

INTRODUCTION

The most common abdominal masses palpable during the newborn period are multicystic dysplastic kidneys, giant hydronephrosis, and infantile forms of polycystic renal disease. True neoplasms of the kidney are distinctly uncommon at this age. The most common renal neoplasm detected in the first month of life is the mesoblastic nephroma.[1] This lesion, also designated fibroma, fibromyoma, fibrosarcoma, leiomyomatous hamartoma, leiomyoma, leiomyosarcoma or fetal hamartoma was almost uniformly described as Wilms' tumor prior to 1966.[2,3] Recently, Bolande has thoroughly reviewed the literature and has emphasized features which distinguish the mesoblastic nephroma from congenital Wilms' tumor.[4]

Nephroblastomatosis has, in the past, also been inappropriately equated with congenital Wilms' tumor. In nephroblastomatosis, usually microscopic but occasionally grossly recognizable foci of undifferentiated tissue are seen in one or both kidneys. Most frequently these are wedge-shaped subcortical or interlobular foci of immature, undifferentiated metanephrogenic tissue in which patches of tubular differentiation may be discernible. Nephroblastomatosis occurs in various autosomal trisomies including trisomy 18[5] and trisomy D, but is perhaps most commonly found in kidneys that harbor a Wilms' tumor. The difficulty of distinguishing nephroblastomatosis associated with Wilms' tumor from a true intrarenal metastasis of a Wilms' tumor is obvious. Lesions of nephroblastomatosis may also occur in the absence of either trisomy or Wilms' tumor. In these circumstances they are more common in newborn infants with congenital malformations than in the general newborn population. Nephroblastomatosis has in the past been designated Wilms' tumor in situ. This is, of course, largely a theoretical concept. Liban and Kozenitsky[6] described nephroblastomatosis in 2 siblings, one of whom had associated mesenchymal hamartomas.

INCIDENCE

Valid ascertainment of the frequency of congenital Wilms' tumors by retrospective review of the literature is obviously impossible. Many reports of presumed congenital Wilms' tumors do not include pathologic illustrations or adequate pathologic descriptions and are, therefore, unacceptable.[7] Several reports with adequate descriptions or illustrations of pathologic findings indicate that the correct diagnosis, in current terminology, should be mesoblastic nephroma.[2,3,8,9]

Fraumeni and Miller[10] reviewed death certificates of 21,659 neonates, from the National Vital Statistics Division of the United States, who died between 1960 and 1964. Of these, 130 died of cancer prior to 28 days of age. There were 9 classified as Wilms' tumor. Legal restrictions precluded access to hospital records for specific

159

pathologic details. In addition, data from death certificates may not reflect the actual frequency of a particular entity since many infants may survive the neonatal period or their tumors may not be recognized until later. A recent review of the National Wilms' Tumor Registry contained approximately 400 or 500 cases; of these, only 1 was in a neonate.[11]

CASE REPORTS

The following two cases include one which has previously been reported in detail.[12] The second was obtained from Dr. Kevin Bove at Cincinnati Children's Hospital.

Case 1.   A 1-day-old male had multiple congenital anomalies including Potter's facies, bilateral flank masses, broad and spadelike hands, polydactyly, webbing of the toes, and bilateral talipes equinovarus deformities without oligohydramnios. Chromosomal analysis showed B-C chromosomal translocation (Figure 1).

Laparotomy revealed unresectable bilateral Wilms' tumor (see renal pathologic description). The infant was given vincristine and dactinomycin. Subse-

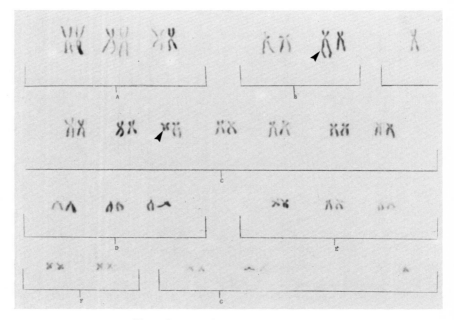

Figure 1.   B-C chromosomal translocation.

quently he developed a bleeding diathesis and leukopenia, and died 8 days postoperatively.

Microscopic examination of renal biopsies obtained at laparotomy showed an undifferentiated anaplastic neoplasm consisting predominantly of spindle-shaped and stellate cells. Occasionally tubular differentiation could be identified (Figure 2). Glomeruloid bodies, neoplastic masses of glomerular epithelial cells recapitulating primitive glomerulogenesis, were numerous.

Case 2.   This full-term male infant weighed 7 lb 12 oz at birth and had a palpable abdominal mass on the left. A left nephrectomy was performed on the second day of life and the tumor weighed 425 g. The child died at 8 days of age with *Escherichia coli* sepsis and renal tubular necrosis. He did not receive radiation therapy or chemotherapy.

Microscopic examination of renal biopsies obtained at laparotomy showed an anaplastic neoplasm consisting predominantly of undifferentiated embryonic stroma of fusiform or stellate cells in which occasional foci of tubular differentiation could be found (Figure 3). Glomeruloid bodies were readily apparent and numerous (Figure 4). Postmortem examination revealed metastatic Wilms' tumor in periaortic nodes.[13]

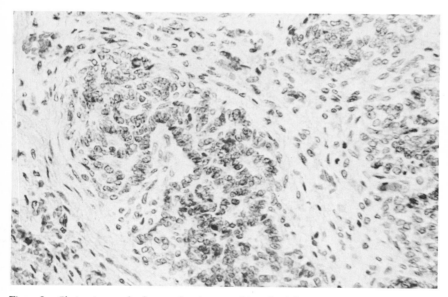

Figure 2.   Photomicrograph of tumor showing area of ductular differentiation in Case 1. The tumor consists of anaplastic, small stellate cells. (H/E stain, 384×).

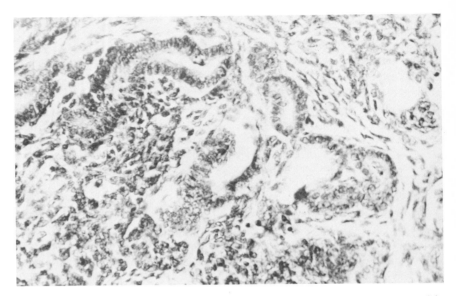

Figure 3. Area of ductular differentiation in Case 2. The otherwise undifferentiated nature of the tumor is evident (below, left). (H/E stain, 384×).

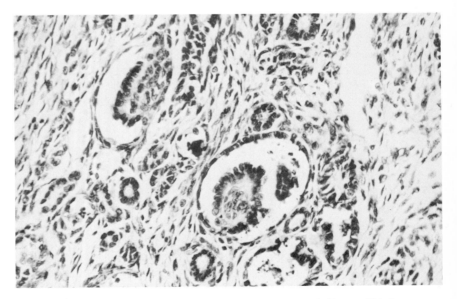

Figure 4. Glomeruloid bodies in the tumor in Case 2. (H/E stain, 384×).

DISCUSSION

True congenital Wilms' tumor is a rare neoplasm but must be included in the differential diagnosis of intrarenal masses in the neonate. Strict pathologic criteria must be adhered to since the prognosis and therapy might be different from that in mesoblastic nephroma, in which nephrectomy alone suffices.

Nephrectomy is obviously indicated in the management of unilateral Wilms' tumor. In those cases with bilateral tumor, unilateral nephrectomy and local excision of the remaining tumor of the opposite kidney should be attempted. In Case 1, the extent of the tumor would have required bilateral nephrectomy and hemodialysis with subsequent renal transplantation.[17] To our knowledge this has not been attempted at this age, although the techniques are now available to accomplish it.

Experience has shown that chemotherapy and radiation therapy, either alone or in combination, are extremely hazardous in infants. The side effects of radiation therapy in children less than 2 years of age are outlined by Dr. Tefft in Chapter 11. These side effects include: (1) severe growth arrest, and (2) secondary malignant tumors.[15] Thus, radiation therapy is not recommended in the neonate.

Our experience and also that of Pochedly[16] attest to the hazard of using vincristine and dactinomycin at this age. We observed leukopenia and overwhelming sepsis; others have observed sudden death in infants given a course of dactinomycin.[17,18] In Case 2, where there were metastases to the periaortic nodes, simple nephrectomy would have seemed to be inadequate therapy. Whether these metastases would regress after excision of the primary tumor, as in some patients with neuroblastoma and retinoblastoma, is unanswerable.

Chromosomal abnormalities described in patients with Wilms' tumor include trisomy 18[19] and pseudohermaphroditism (XX/XY mosaicism).[20] After statistical analysis of their own cases, Knudson and Strong[21] concluded that bilateral Wilms' tumors are likely to be familial and display a pattern consistent with autosomal dominant inheritance (see Chapter 4). Chromosomal instability occurs in cells of patients with such genetic disorders as Bloom's syndrome, ataxia telangiectasia, Fanconi's anemia, and xeroderma pigmentosum. These disorders are also prone to the development of cancer and the frequency is greater than that which would be expected by chance alone. Ladda et al.[22] were able to detect a small deletion on chromosome 8 in a child with aniridia and Wilms' tumor, using a high-resolution microscope scanning system coupled to a computer. In Case 1 there is also a translocation between the long arm of a B chromosome and the long arm of a C chromosome. Banding techniques were inconclusive in an attempt to identify the specific chromosome involved. These findings may be important to our understanding of the mechanism of carcinogenesis or may represent an isolated combination of chromosomal abnormalities and Wilms' tumor.

We have described 2 patients with true congenital Wilms' tumor, one with bilateral involvement, multiple congenital anomalies and B-C chromosomal translocation and the other with metastatic involvement of the periaortic nodes. Neither survived, and chemotherapy may have contributed to Case 1's demise.

The improved survival rate reported for Wilms' tumor under 1 year of age may be partially based upon the unintentional inclusion of cases of mesoblastic nephroma among the infants studied. Thus it appears that we must reappraise our present understanding of true congenital Wilms' tumor with respect to treatment, survival, and prognosis.

SUMMARY

It is imperative to adhere to the strict pathologic criteria of Wilms' tumor prior to institution of definitive therapy. It is apparent even from the recent literature that confusion persists between identification of congenital Wilms' tumor and its benign counterpart, mesoblastic nephroma, despite the detailed description by Bolande[4] that differentiates these neoplasms. Therefore the therapeutic implications and prognosis must be reassessed in view of the renewed understanding that distinguishes these neoplasms.

Careful chromosome analysis might be performed prospectively in patients with Wilms' tumors at facilities that are equipped and utilize the sophisticated techniques of chromosomal banding coupled to a computer, as described by Ladda et al.[22] The purpose is to establish whether or not the recent reports of chromosomal aberrations are coincidental or have a permissive role which allows malignant neoplasms to develop in these individuals. The rarity of congenital Wilms' tumor would require a cooperative effort of several centers prior to answering many of these questions.

REFERENCES

1. Bolande, R.: Benignity of neonatal tumors and concepts of cancer regression in early life. *Am. J. Dis. Child.* **122**:12, 1971.
2. Baert, L., Verduyn, H., and Vereecken, R.: Wilms' tumor; a report of 51 histologically proven cases. *J. Urol.* **96**:871, 1966.
3. DeNicola, R. R., and Armstrong, T. H.: Neonatal tumors of the kidney. *Am. J. Surg.* **94**:502, 1957.
4. Bolande, R.: Congenital mesoblastic nephroma of infancy. In *Perspectives in Pediatric Pathology*, vol. I, Year Book Medical Publishers, Chicago, 1973. p. 227.
5. Bove, K. E., Koffler, H., and McAdams, A. J.: Nodular renal blastema; Definition and possible significance. *Cancer* **24**:323, 1969.
6. Liban, E., and Kozenitsky, I. L.: Metanephric hamartomas and nephroblastomatosis in siblings. *Cancer* **25**:885, 1970.

7. Longino, L. A., and Martin, L. A.: Abdominal masses in the newborn infant. *Pediatrics* **21**:596, 1958.

8. Walker, P., and Richard, G. A.: Fetal hamartomas of the kidney. *J. Urol.* **110**:352, 1973.

9. Wright, E. S.: Congenital Wilms' tumour; case report. *Br. J. Urol.* **42**:270, 1970.

10. Fraumeni, J. F., Jr., and Miller, R. W.: Cancer deaths in the newborn. *Am. J. Dis. Child.* **117**:186, 1969.

11. Beckwith, J.: Personal communication, 1974.

12. Giangiacomo, J., Penchansky, L., Monteleone, P. L., and Thompson, J.: Bilateral neonatal Wilms' tumor with B-C chromosomal translocation. *J. Pediatr.* **86**:98, 1975.

13. Bove, K.: Personal communication, 1974.

14. DeLorimier, A. A., Belzer, F. O., Kounty, S. L., and Kushner, J. H.: Simultaneous bilateral nephrectomy and renal allotransplantation for bilateral Wilms' tumor. *Surgery* **64**:850, 1968.

15. Tefft, M., Vawter, G. F., and Mitus, A.: Second primary neoplasms in children. *Am. J. Roentgenol.* **103**:800, 1968.

16. Pochedly, C., Collucci, J. A., Kenigsberg, K., and Loesevitz, A.: Hazard of chemotherapy in congenital Wilms' tumor. *J. Pediatr.* **79**:708, 1971.

17. Kay, S., Pratt, C., and Salzberg, A.: Hamartoma (leiomyomatous type) of the kidney. *Cancer* **19**:1825, 1966.

18. Young, D., and Williams, D.: Malignant renal tumours in infancy and childhood. *Br. J. Hosp. Med.* **2**:741, 1969.

19. Gieser, C. F., and Schindler, A. M.: Long term survival in a male with 18-trisomy syndrome and Wilms' tumor. *Pediatrics* **44**:111, 1969.

20. Denys, P., Mal Vaux, P., Van den Berghe, H., et al.: Association d'un syndrome anatomopathologique de pseudohermaphrodisme masculin, d'une tumeur de Wilms', d'une nephropathie parenchymateuse et d'un mosaicisme XX/XY. *Arch. Fr. Pediatr.* **24**:729, 1967.

21. Knudson, A. G., Jr., and Strong, L. C.: Mutation and cancer: a model for Wilms' tumor of the kidney. *J. Natl. Cancer Inst.* **48**:313, 1972.

22. Ladda, R., Atkins, L., and Littlefield, J.: Computer-assisted analysis of chromosomal abnormalities; detection of a deletion in aniridia/Wilms' tumor syndrome. *Science* **185**:784, 1974.

CHAPTER ELEVEN

Surgical Treatment of Wilms' Tumor

ALFRED A. DE LORIMIER, M.D.

Pediatric Surgical Service
Associate Professor
Department of Surgery
School of Medicine
University of California
San Francisco, California

CONTENTS

INTRODUCTION

The extraordinary improvement in the results of treatment of Wilms' tumor has made it a model in the management of many other malignancies. In 1927 the cure rate for Wilms' tumor was only 9%.[1] From 1941 to 1959 several series of children with Wilms' tumors were reported in which nephrectomy alone, usually performed through a retroperitoneal flank incision, achieved a cure rate of 13 to 23%.[2,3] In 1950 Gross and Neuhauser[4] described their technique of combined transperitoneal nephrectomy with postoperative radiotherapy and reported a survival rate of 47%. In 1955 Farber[5] noted that dactinomycin produced significant regression in a case of metastatic Wilms' tumor, and in 1966 he described a series of 68 children who had nephrectomy, radiotherapy, and prophylactic dactinomycin, resulting in a 2-year survival rate of 80%. Since then numerous reports have appeared documenting the efficacy of dactinomycin, vincristine, or both chemotherapeutic agents given together in addition to surgery and radiotherapy.

It is important to recognize that permanent control of clinically obvious metastases is rarely obtained by using chemotherapeutic agents alone.[6] Dramatic regression of an established primary or metastatic tumor follows chemotherapy in 70 to 80% of cases, but after a period of time and with repeated courses of chemotherapy the tumor mass will regrow unless either radiotherapy or surgical resection is added to the therapeutic regimen.[7-9] Presently available chemotherapeutic agents are most effective in eradicating microscopic foci of tumor.[10] This concept is apparent when comparing the incidence of metastatic tumor following nephrectomy with and without chemotherapy. In children who were treated for primary Wilms' tumor, had no metastases initially, and received no chemotherapy, 45 to 57% subsequently developed metastases.[10-14] The use of prophylactic dactinomycin in a comparable group of children reduced the incidence of late metastases to 10 to 20%.[5,10,11,12,14,15]

The current enthusiasm for chemotherapy in the treatment of Wilms' tumor may adversely overshadow the importance of meticulous surgical technique as an integral part of the treatment to achieve high curability. Just as antibiotics were once thought to make careful antiseptic technique in surgery less important, chemotherapy of tumors might be considered sufficient to overcome careless surgical excision of the tumor. The surgical procedure must be performed meticulously to prevent rupture or dissemination via lymphatics and venous drainage. In the Children's Cancer Study Group A report, several patients were excluded from statistical evaluation because of operative spillage of the tumor.[15] Cassady et al.[16] reported on 20 of 156 children in whom spillage of tumor occurred at operation. In a cooperative study by the Société Internationale Oncologie Pediatrique, intraoperative rupture of the tumor occurred in 30% of 43 patients who had received no preoperative radiation therapy.[17] Although Wilms' tumor can be cured in spite of operative rupture of the tumor, postoperative recurrence and death is the more common sequel.[16-18] The operative procedure must be conducted with the recognition that many of these tumors are extremely friable and have extended through the capsule of the kidney, and that one-third have spread to adjacent lymph nodes and/or into the renal veins, and that extension down the ureter with implantation into the lower urinary tract occasionally occurs.

Surgical excision of metastases is an important adjunct in treatment. Surgical resection of metastatic tumor will have to be considered with respect to the clinical circumstances, the extent of the disease, the rate of tumor growth, and the sensitivity of the tumor to chemotherapy and radiation therapy.

PREOPERATIVE CONSIDERATIONS

Wilms' tumor is a very rapidly growing neoplasm, and the principle of complete diagnostic evaluation within 24 hours after discovery of the mass is warranted. Diagnostic procedures such as intravenous pyelogram (IVP), chest roentgenograms, tomograms, liver scan, abdominal ultrasonogram, and renal arteriogram are discussed by Dr. Young (Chapter 7). Retrograde pyelograms are not indicated, even when there is nonvisualization of the kidney on IVP. The affected kidney will not visualize on IVP in 15 to 30% of patients with Wilms' tumor, because the tumor has grown into the renal vein or into the renal pelvis and down the ureter.[13,19] Preliminary data from the National Wilms' Tumor Study indicate that 36% of 289 patients had tumor extension into the renal pelvis or calices.[20] The potential for implantation of tumor into the lower urinary tract in these cases must be considered.[21] If the nature of the mass must be clarified by further studies, an ultrasonogram and renal arteriogram will provide details that will influence treatment better than retrograde urography.

Evaluation of the bloodclotting mechanism is important, because disseminated intravascular coagulopathy has been described.[22] Abnormality in the clotting mechanism may be important to recognize, not necessarily to postpone the operation, but to be prepared for exchange transfusion with fresh blood, fresh frozen plasma, or platelets.

An associated illness may require delay in nephrectomy. Hypertension is frequent in children with Wilms' tumor and is occasionally accompanied by congestive heart failure. Impaired respiration from a large tumor may produce pneumonia which must be treated first. Occasionally, extensive lung metastases may impair pulmonary function and require preoperative chemotherapy and radiotherapy. The objective of the delay is to return the child to a state of health in which operative removal of the primary tumor will be followed by minimal postoperative morbidity. The time for the operation should depend upon the clinical status of the patient. Preoperative chemotherapy to the point of severe toxicity or the preoperative use of radiotherapy to an arbitrary dose must be avoided so that nephrectomy may be done without delay. Chemotherapy and radiotherapy can be easily resumed soon after excision of the primary tumor mass.

An enormous tumor may require preoperative radiotherapy and chemotherapy to reduce its size, facilitate operative removal, and minimize the risk of disseminating metastases.[23.] There has been concern that metastases occur if surgical resection is delayed to reduce the size of the tumor. However, several reports published prior to the use of chemotherapy indicate improved survival in those patients with large tumors who were treated by irradiation therapy preoperatively as well as postoperatively.[3,17,23,24] Preoperative radiation therapy will allow an assessment of the radiosensitivity of the tumor. Chemotherapy has also been used to reduce the size of the tumor, but probably the combination of chemotherapy and irradiation is most effective. The timing of the operation is selected according to the response of the tumor, but it probably should not be delayed beyond 10 days. If there is little regression in the size of the mass within 7 to 10 days, the tumor is probably radioresistant and surgical resection should be done.

Normal saline enemas should be given preoperatively to those children who have a large, aggressively-growing tumor which may have locally invaded the colon and its mesentery. In these instances resection of the bowel may be necessary, and a mechanical bowel cleansing would obviate the need for a colostomy instead of primary anastomosis.

OPERATIVE TECHNIQUE

Following the induction of endotracheal anesthesia, a cutdown or large-bore plastic cannula should be placed in one of the upper extremities or in the superior vena cava. It may be necessary to clamp the inferior vena cava, and large volumes of blood or fluid replacement may become sequestered instead of rapidly replenishing blood volume if the lower extremities are cannulated. The adequacy of blood volume replacement can be monitored by measuring a rise in right atrial pressure and by sampling blood from the right heart and aorta for measurement of blood gas and pH. Metabolic acidosis and a large arteriovenous oxygen difference indicate inadequate tissue perfusion from hypovolemia or heart failure. We usually avoid placing a Foley catheter in the bladder because of the risk of producing pyelonephritis in the remaining kidney. However, if an extensive dissection is anticipated, a urinary catheter will help monitor perfusion of the uninvolved kidney by continuously recording the volume of urinary output during the course of the procedure.

The chest and the abdomen should be sterilely prepared for a large, upper-pole tumor that may require elongation of the abdominal incision into the thorax. A *long* transverse incision in the upper abdomen should extend for the complete length of both costal margins. Children who have been referred to us because of intraoperative spillage of tumor have invariably had small incisions. A long incision allows extensive dissection of the tumor without having to retract or rotate the mass with the risk of rupturing the tumor or disseminating metastases.

Initially the liver and retroperitoneal lymph nodes are examined for evidence of metastases. The other kidney should be carefully examined to rule out possible bilateral involvement. This may require mobilization of the colon and kidney so that all surfaces can be examined.

For right-sided tumors the cecum, ascending and right transverse colon, and for left-sided tumors the descending and left transverse colon must be mobilized beyond the midline to gain access to the retroperitoneum.

Biopsy of a renal tumor is indicated if there is a compelling reason to save the kidney or if there is a significant possibility that the mass is benign. The most important principle in removal of nephroblastoma is wide en bloc resection of the tumor, including the involved adjacent organs and regional lymph nodes. The dissection requires knowledge of the lymph drainage of the kidney and the anatomy of Gerota's fascia. Martin and Reyes,[25] from Rouviere's work, showed that there are three lymphatic pathways from the kidney to central nodes. The anterior one-third of the kidney drains by way of lymphatic channels anterior to the renal vein. The middle third of the kidney drains via lymphatic vessels between the renal artery and vein, and the posterior third of the kidney drains through lymphatics posterior to the renal artery. These lymphatic channels diverge to lymph nodes along the aorta on the left side and the vena cava on the right (Figure 1). Some of these lymphatics course directly to the lymph nodes between the aorta and vena cava. The para-aortic and para-vena cava nodes also drain into the nodes between the aorta and the vena cava, and from there the lymphatics course to the cisterna chyli and the thoracic duct to empty into the subclavian veins. The nodes that concern the surgeon are distributed from the diaphragm to the level of the inferior mesenteric artery.

Gerota's fascia, or the renal fascia, forms a natural envelope around the kidneys, adrenal glands, ureters, and lymphatics draining the kidney.[26] Gerota's fascia develops between the transversalis fascia and the peritoneum. It splits into an anterior and posterior sheath lateral to the quadratus lumborum muscles to encompass the kidneys. Medially, the posterior sheath of Gerota's fascia fuses with the transversalis fascia and becomes attached to the anterior ligament of the vertebrae. The anterior sheath of Gerota's fascia extends across the midline anterior to the aorta and the vena cava. Between the anterior and posterior leaves of the renal fascia there is a variable amount of fat, numerous lymphatic channels, and plexuses of autonomic nerve fibers from the celiac ganglia. When the dissection for radical nephrectomy is performed outside of Gerota's fascia, a readily identifiable plane will facilitate en bloc resection of the tumor and adjacent lymphatics.

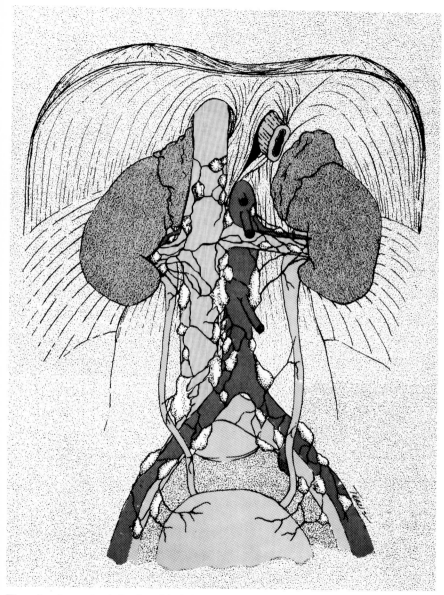

Figure 1. Anatomic relationship of the kidneys and their lymphatic drainage to the aorta, vena cava, diaphragm, and posterior abdominal muscles.

The dissection should begin medially between the aorta and the inferior vena cava. The retroperitoneum, the contained vessels, lymphatics, and autonomic fibers are divided between clamps and tied. This dissection should extend posteriorly to the vertebrae between the aorta and the vena cava from the level of the superior mesenteric artery and diaphragm to the aortic bifurcation. The renal vein and artery are divided as early as possible in the procedure. The perivascular plane of Leriche allows easy mobilization of the retroperitoneal lymphatics off the major vessels. The dissection is continued laterally and posteriorly adjacent to the aorta or the vena cava to divide the posterior sheath of Gerota's fascia adjacent to the vertebrae and psoas muscle. Usually division of the lumbar vessels facilitates the development of the plane behind the posterior sheath of Gerota's fascia. In the course of this dissection the superior mesenteric and celiac arteries must be identified and carefully preserved.

The renal veins and the vena cava must be carefully palpated for evidence of tumor extension. Engorged retroperitoneal collateral venous channels indicate obstruction of the renal vein. Early in the course of the procedure, the renal vein should be divided at the junction with the inferior vena cava. However, if there is tumor in the vena cava, the length of its involvement must be determined, assessing whether the tumor affects the contralateral renal venous drainage, hepatic venous channels, or whether it extends into the right atrium. It is important to cross-clamp the vena cava above the level of tumor extension to prevent embolus into the pulmonary artery with the possibility of sudden death. Usually the tumor thrombus is not adherent to the vena cava and, after isolating the involved segment with vascular clamps, it can be extracted intact. If the tumor has grown as far as the intrahepatic portion of the vena cava, the abdominal incision has to be extended into the right thorax to assess whether tumor exists in the right atrium. It is possible to clamp the atrium, avoiding the sinus nodes, and extract the tumor by an atriotomy. Arrangements for cardiopulmonary bypass may be required to open the right atrium.[27] However, removal of tumor from the vena cava or right atrium should be deferred to the last stage of the operation, so that when the tumor is removed it can be walled off to prevent implantation of tumor cells into the abdominal or thoracic cavity.

If the tumor is adherent to the vena cava, that segment of the vein may have to be removed. The inferior vena cava can be resected in children without congestion in the lower extremities, because of extensive collateral venous return to the heart. The left renal vein can be divided without reestablishing continuity to the vena cava, because of the effective collateral drainage adjacent to the left renal hilus. Venous collateral drainage from the right kidney is less well developed, and sudden occlusion of the right renal vein may result in infarction of the kidney. It is possible that gradual obstruction of the right renal vein by tumor thrombus arising from the left kidney might stimulate adequate collateral venous drainage from the right kidney. Prosthetic replacement of the vena cava or renal veins is probably not effective, because it would thrombose in this low pressure system.

If the retrohepatic portion of the vena cava contains densely adherent tumor, it is not possible to resect that portion of the vein. Every effort should be made to extract the tumor from the vein, since cure depends upon a tumor that will respond to postoperative radiotherapy and chemotherapy.

Tumor thrombus in the inferior vena cava probably should not be treated preoperatively with radiotherapy and chemotherapy, because this technique will probably produce dense adherence of the tumor to the vein wall and compromise surgical removal. Whenever tumor has been removed from the vena cava, postoperative irradiation of the vena cava and also the bed of the kidney is indicated.

In almost one-half of cases the tumor has extended through the renal capsule and Gerota's fascia to become adherent to or invade adjacent structures such as the adrenal gland, pancreas, duodenum, spleen, liver, diaphragm, back muscles, and colon. The surgeon must be prepared to resect these structures en bloc with the tumor (Figures 2,3). Clinical judgment is required to decide whether a safe plane can be developed between an adherent organ without entering the tumor. Operative rupture of the tumor occurs not only from inappropriate retraction on the tumor but also from failure to remove the tumor with a wide margin including the involved adjacent structures. The entire ureter should be removed down to the base of the bladder (Figure 4). Usually the ovarian and testicular vessels and the lumbar sympathetic ganglia are removed to accomplish the necessary wide resection required. During the course of the procedure manipulation and retraction of the tumor is avoided until the last portion of the procedure, for most nephroblastomas are very friable, and pressure on the tumor will massage malignant cells into the lymphatic and venous channels or rupture the capsule resulting in direct implantation of the tumor. The dissection posterior to Gerota's fascia usually begins medially, and a good plane over the psoas and quadratus muscles can be developed. It may be necessary to resect part of the diaphragm, transversus abdominis, quadratus lumborum, or psoas muscles if tumor has grown beyond the posterior sheath of Gerota's fascia.

After the mass is removed, metal clips may be placed in areas of the tumor bed that need localization for postoperative radiation therapy. If there is any leakage of lymph, the source should be identified and ligated.

Meticulous attention to the technical details in removal of the primary tumor is the first step toward achieving cure.

TREATMENT OF METASTATIC WILMS' TUMOR

While patients with Wilms' tumor are being followed, they must be carefully reevaluated at least every 3 months for a period of 3 years for evidence of recurrent or metastatic tumor. Routine blood count, platelet count, chest x-ray, liver scan, and IVP must be repeated to screen the patient for possible recurrent tumor. If

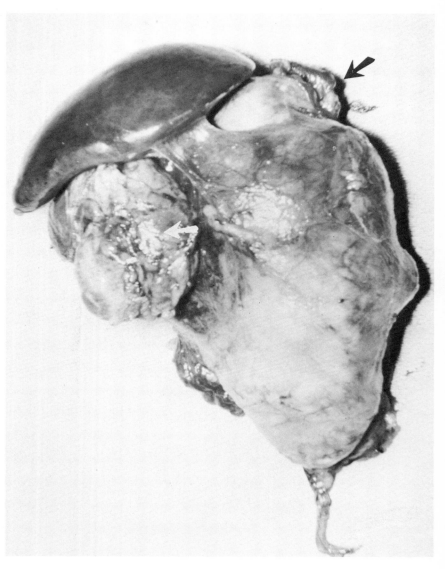

Figure 2. Wilms' tumor resected en bloc with spleen, diaphragm (black arrow), tail of pancreas (white arrow), and ureter.

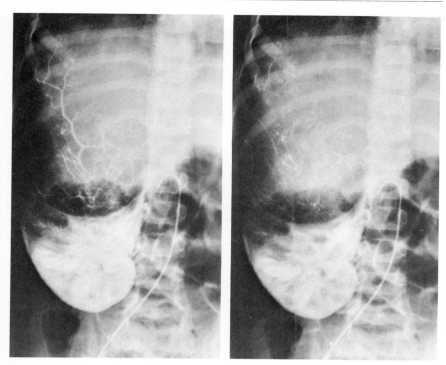

Figure 3.   Arteriogram showing large, upper pole Wilms' tumor of right kidney invading the liver. En bloc resection of the tumor required removal of a portion of the diaphragm and posterior segment of the right lobe of the liver with the kidney.

metastases appear, intraabdominal recurrence or extension of tumor into the inferior vena cava must be considered and may warrant an inferior vena cavogram and "second look" exploratory laparotomy.

At initial diagnosis, metastases will be found in the lung in 15 to 30% of patients and in the liver in 5 to 10% of cases.[5,12,16,19,28] Those children who do not have obvious metastases at first diagnosis, and who receive repeated prophylactic courses of chemotherapy, will subsequently develop metastases in 20 to 30% of cases.[11,14,15,16] In the older series of children who developed metastatic Wilms' tumor, metastases were present initially or became evident within 6 months in 70 to 80% of cases.[19,29] Metastases appeared between 6 months to 12 months in 15% and beyond 1 year in 15% of the children.[19,29] The lung accounted for 60 to 75% of the recurrent lesions, and 24 to 36% of these children developed tumor in other organs as well.[16,19] These data included patients treated by a variety of regimens, and most of them had not had dactinomycin or vincristine. In a more recent evaluation, the efficacy of single-course versus multiple-course dactinomycin was

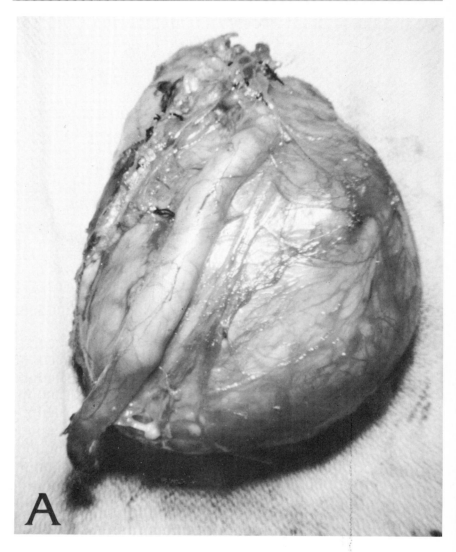

compared in children with completely resected Stage I tumors.[15] Of 28 patients given a single course of dactinomycin, 12 developed metastases confined to the lung and 4 had extrapulmonary tumor. Of 25 children receiving multiple courses of dactinomycin, only 1 had isolated pulmonary metastases and 6 developed extrapulmonary spread. The current use of multiple courses of two or more chemotherapeutic agents may alter the incidence and distribution of metastases to a greater extent than dactinomycin alone has in the past.

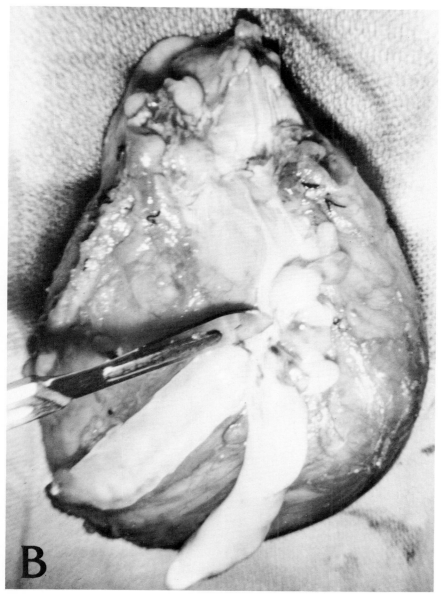

Figures 4(A) and (B). Wilms' tumor growing into the renal pelvis and down the ureter.

Multiple metastases in the lung and/or liver or in anatomic sites that are not readily accessible for complete surgical resection should be treated initially with radiation therapy in addition to chemotherapy. At the University of California, San Francisco, lung metastases are treated according to a dose schedule derived by Wara et al.,[30] based on the incidence of radiation pneumonitis. The usual schedule is 1500 rads in 10 fractions to both entire lung fields. These radiation dosage schedules are based on the simultaneous use of dactinomycin and its potentiation of the radiation effect. Approximately 40 to 60% of patients treated with this regimen have gained permanent control of their pulmonary lesions.[30]

Whole lung tomograms should be performed to identify the presence or absence of persistent tumor. If there is evidence of persistent tumor we prefer surgical resection of the residual disease, even when multiple or bilateral lesions or both are present. Some have advocated a second course of irradiation using portals that only encompass residual tumor. The intent of using small portals is to localize destruction of pulmonary parenchyma to the volume of lung encompassed by the radiation ports. However, second courses of radiation therapy usually fail.[16,31,32] More lung parenchyma is destroyed by the radiation therapy than that required for surgical excision, because unaffected areas and lobes of the lung overlap those areas that contain tumor and they are included in the treatment field.

Wohl et al.[32] performed pulmonary function studies on 20 children, 7 to 14 years following treatment for Wilms' tumor by nephrectomy, postoperative radiotherapy to the abdomen, and dactinomycin. Of these children, 8 who had no pulmonary metastases served as controls and they had total lung capacity (TLC), vital capacity (VC), functional residual capacity (FRC), and diffusing capacity (DlCO) more than 90% of predicted normal values. Six children who developed pulmonary metastases received only one course of radiation therapy to both lungs of 850 to 1250 rads. In these 6 patients the TLC, VC, FRC and DlCO was diminished to approximately 72% of normal. Four children were treated by a second course of radiation therapy of 1250 to 1900 rads, and they required a subsequent pulmonary resection. The TLC, VC, FRC and DlCO of these children were reduced to 30 to 60% of normal. Two children had surgical resection of persistent tumor following the initial course of pulmonary irradiation, and their lung function tests were equivalent to the group that had been treated by only one course of radiation therapy. The authors concluded that some pulmonary fibrosis might have occurred, but radiation primarily affected the development of alveoli, and not the airways, and produced a decrease in the size of the lung and chest wall.

Most pulmonary metastases occur in the periphery of the lung parenchyma, and simple but wide wedge resection is readily accomplished. Occasionally a more centrally placed lesion would require segmental resection or lobectomy. With surgical excision, a smaller volume of lung is sacrificed, and morbidity is minimal—the average postoperative hospital stay is 5 days (Figures 5,6).

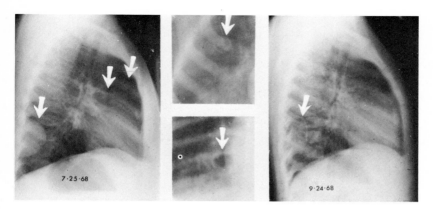

Figure 5. Multiple metastatic Wilms' tumors in the lung. These lesions responded to 1500 rads radiation (plus dactinomycin and vincristine) by cavitating, but they recurred within 3 months. The patient is alive without recurrence 7 years after thoracotomy and wedge resection of the metastases.

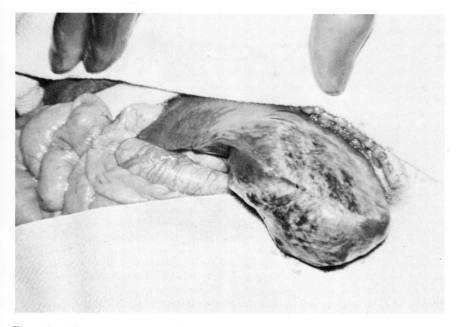

Figure 6. Solitary metastasis in the liver was excised by wedge resection and the whole liver was irradiated with 2500 rads. The patient is alive without recurrence 6 years later.

The role of surgical resection initially, rather than radiation therapy, in the treatment of solitary metastatic lesions will require continual assessment. In older series, approximately 60% of the pulmonary metastases were multiple and most of these appeared bilaterally.[29] The frequency of apparent solitary pulmonary lesions eventually becoming multiple has not been well documented. Monson et al.[31] described 11 children who seemed to have solitary metastases, but 6 developed other metastatic lesions. Kilman et al.[33] reviewed the reported cases of pulmonary resection for metastatic Wilms' tumor and described apparent cure in 21 of 31 patients. Only 8 of these children developed additional new lung recurrences and 5 were long-term survivors after a second or third pulmonary resection.[33] Repeated courses of dactinomycin have changed the incidence of pulmonary metastasis, and it remains to be seen if the pattern of solitary or multiple pulmonary lesions changes.[15] The role of surgical resection initially for solitary lesions will probably be decided on an individual basis until more information is available about the natural history of these lesions when treated with current chemotherapy programs. Although repeated courses of dactinomycin reduced the incidence of pulmonary metastases, the survival rate of the children who had a single course or multiple courses of dactinomycin was the same. This was because the subsequent treatment of the pulmonary metastases was so effective with the use of additional chemotherapy, radiotherapy, and surgical excision.[15]

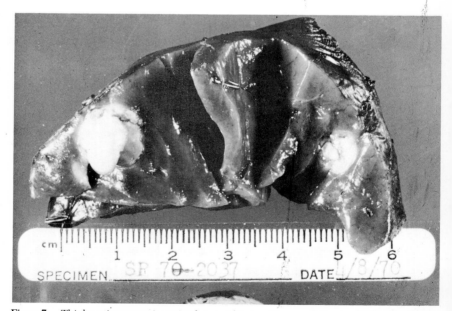

Figure 7.   This hepatic metastasis persisted on serial isotope liver scan following 2500 rads radiation. A right posterior hepatic resection was performed, and the patient is alive without recurrence 5 years postoperatively.

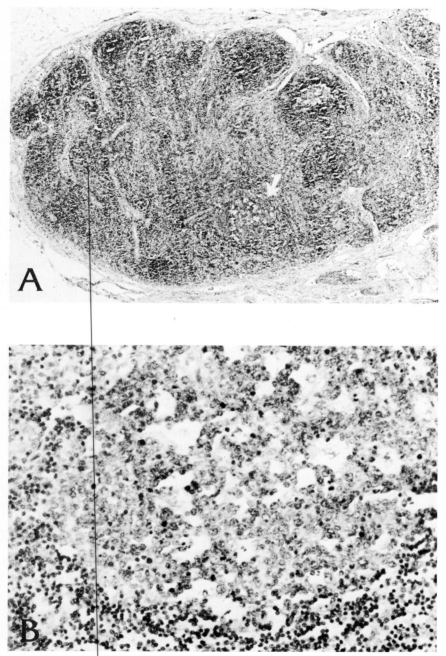

Figure 8. A small focus of metastatic Wilms' tumor (arrow) in a normal-appearing lymph node between the aorta and the vena cava. (H/E stain. Magnification in A is 27.60×, in B 172.50×).

The liver is the second most frequent site of metastasis.[19,28] Follow-up evaluation of the patient must include a liver scan at least every 3 months within the first 3 years to detect these lesions. When the liver is involved, metastases are commonly present in multiple areas within the liver and in extrahepatic sites.[16] False-positive liver scans are common, particularly following chemotherapy and radiotherapy to the liver. Exploratory laparotomy and, preferably, excisional biopsy might be necessary for questionable lesions. Hepatic metastases should be treated with radiation therapy and continuation of the chemotherapy. A dose of 2000 to 2500 rads in 15 fractions should be delivered to the entire liver.[30]

Impaired hepatic function produces exaggerated systemic toxicity from chemotherapeutic agents. Therefore, subsequent courses of dactinomycin or vincristine will have to be modified at the time hepatic function is depressed following removal of a significant portion of the liver or hepatic irradiation.[34]

If a left nephrectomy has been performed, the right kidney should be shielded to prevent radiation nephritis. It is possible to relocate the right kidney in a position outside the radiation field, but usually alteration of radiation techniques such as the use of lateral portals can be accomplished to deliver the dose necessary to eradicate hepatic metastases.

If isotope scans demonstrate one or more persistent defects in the liver 3 months after radiation therapy, and no other metastases are evident, exploratory laparotomy and excision of the residual lesions is indicated.[35,36] The surgical procedure may consist of simple wedge excision of a peripheral lesion or a hepatic lobectomy may be indicated for more centrally placed tumors (Figures 7,8). There is no current information about the efficacy of cannulating the hepatic artery for perfusion of antitumor agents in Wilms' tumor. When a significant volume of the liver has been removed, the "regenerating" residual liver may be severely affected if dactinomycin and/or hepatic irradiation are administered within 6 weeks of the hepatic resection.[34,36] Therefore liver function tests and repeated liver isotope scans will be necessary to detect the occurrence of full hepatic regeneration. More aggressive management of hepatic metastases, including surgical resection, should be encouraged to achieve greater curability of these tumors.

DISCUSSION

At present many surgeons resect only those lymph nodes immediately adjacent to the kidney hilus or "berry-pick" obviously enlarged nodes. They would disagree with the need for wide en bloc lymph node dissection as described here. Most infants with tumors confined to the renal parenchyma probably do not require an extensive lymphadenectomy since local recurrence is very rare in this age group. However, the treatment and prognosis in children depends heavily upon accurately staging the extent of the tumor (see Table 1, Chapter 11). Radiation therapy to the tumor bed and central chain of nodes is unnecessary for patients who have Stage I (group I) tumors with no lymph node involvement, but it is imperative for those who have lymphatic metastases. Therefore recognition of lymphatic spread of tumor requires excision of all the nodes that drain the kidney.

Lymph node metastases have been reported in 12 to 35% of patients with Wilms' tumor.[25] During the past 8 years we have performed the thorough periaortic node dissection en bloc with the kidney and tumor as described here. The resected specimens contained 11 to 26 lymph nodes. Of 21 patients, 6 had lymph node metastases, and in 3 patients the more central nodes were involved when the hilar nodes were not.

The pathologist also has an important responsibility in defining the stage of the disease. He must locate and examine all of the resected lymph nodes, because metastases can be microscopic in size in otherwise normal-appearing nodes (Figure 8). In the National Wilms' Tumor Study 313 cases in Stages I, II and III have been studied, and the status of the lymph nodes was not recorded in 35% either because the nodes were not removed, not examined, or not reported upon.[20] Preliminary data from the National Wilms' Tumor Study, comparing children with Stage I tumor who had postoperative radiation or no radiation therapy, suggests a higher incidence of intraabdominal recurrence in the nonirradiated group.[20] If recurrence is truly more common in the nonirradiated group, the implication is that they were improperly staged and treated because of failure to resect lymph nodes which contained tumor. Whether radical en bloc lymphadenectomy will favorably influence the prognosis, in addition to irradiation and chemotherapy, remains to be seen. Only cooperative prospective analyses such as the National Wilms' Tumor Study will provide answers to these important issues.

Surgical resection of solitary metastases would be the procedure of choice if it were possible to identify truly solitary lesions in the lung or liver. Factors which might identify this group of patients include the age of the patient, extension of tumor in the renal vein and/or lymph node metastases, and growth rate and histology of the tumor. It will be necessary to correlate these factors with the clinical course of the disease for some time before reliable predictions will be available.

Collins et al.[37] described the relatively constant growth rate of a number of tumors, and they developed a method of identifying the time required for a tumor mass to double in size. Recently Joseph et al.[38] calculated the tumor-doubling time of a variety of neoplasms that had metastasized to the lung, and they suggested that the prognosis and results of metastatic resection could be correlated with the tumor-doubling time. Patients with a tumor-doubling time of less than 20 days had an interval of 4.8 months between control of the primary tumor and the appearance of metastases, and all of these patients died. Patients with a tumor-doubling time of > 40 days had an average interval of 29.5 months between treatment of their primary tumor and the appearance of pulmonary metastases. All of these patients were long-term survivors after removal of solitary or multiple bilateral metastases.

This information may not be suitable for evaluation of children with metastatic Wilms' tumor. Treatment of metastases should not be delayed to watch the rate of tumor growth. The tumor-doubling time would have to be identified indirectly by noting the interval of time required for metastatic lesions to become clinically evident. Dactinomycin does not seem to alter the interval between the treatment of primary Wilms' tumor and the appearance of its metastases,[11,12] but the combination of dactinomycin and vincristine may do so. Moreover, the prognosis following resection of metastatic Wilms' tumor seems to be better in those patients who develop metastases early rather than late after control of the primary tumor. In the review by Kilman et al.[33] the average interval for metastases to appear was 7 months in the survivors and 14 months in those patients who died.

Bilateral pulmonary metastases should be no deterrent to surgical resection.[33] More aggressive management of hepatic metastases, including surgical resection, should be encouraged to achieve greater curability of these tumors.

CONCLUSION

The treatment of Wilms' tumor requires a closely integrated team of surgeon, radiotherapist, chemotherapist, radiologist, and pathologist. Each patient should be reviewed by the group at frequent intervals, and the treatment plan should be formulated by an appraisal of the extent of the disease and the advantages and limitations of the available therapeutic modalities.

The surgical member of the team must accomplish a wide en bloc resection of the primary tumor, using gentle and meticulous technique to prevent rupture or dissemination of the tumor via venous and lymphatic channels. He must work with the pathologist to help stage the extent of the tumor, and he must add a surgical perspective to the overall assessment of the patient.

The treatment of metastases to the lungs, liver, brain, or bone is primarily with x-ray therapy plus dactinomycin and vincristine. Metastatic tumor that persists after radiation therapy should be surgically removed. The role of surgical resection of apparently solitary metastases initially, in lieu of irradiation, requires further clarification and will have to be individualized. The presence of multiple metastases should not be a deterrent to surgical resection.

At present it is clear from a number of reported series that the best results in the treatment of Wilms' tumor are in centers that have a team who care for significant numbers of patients with these rare tumors.[5,12,16,36]

REFERENCES

1. Wollstein, M.: Renal neoplasms in young children. *Arch. Pathol.* **3**:1–13, 1927.

2. Ladd, W. E., and White, R. R.: Embryoma of the kidney (Wilms' tumor). *JAMA* **117**:1858–1862, 1941.

3. Abeshouse, B. S.: The management of Wilms' tumor as determined by national survey and review of the literature. *J. Urol.* **77**:792–813, 1957.

4. Gross, R. E., and Neuhauser, E. B. D.: Treatment of mixed tumors of the kidney in childhood. *Pediatrics* **6**:843–852, 1950.

5. Farber, S.: Chemotherapy in the treatment of leukemia and Wilms' tumor. *JAMA* **198**:826–836, 1966.

6. Maier, J. G., and Harshaw, W. G.: Treatment and prognosis in Wilms' tumor. a study of 51 cases with special reference to the role of actinomycin D. *Cancer* **20**:96–102, 1967.

7. Tan, C. T. C., Dargeon, H. W., and Bunchenal, J. H.: The effect of actinomycin D on cancer in childhood. *Pediatrics* **24**:544–561, 1959.

8. Shaw, R. K., Moore, E. W., Mueller, P. S., Frei, E., and Watkin, D. M.: The effect of actinomycin D on childhood neoplasms. *Am. J. Dis. Child.* **99**:96–103, 1960.

9. Sullivan, M. P., Sutow, W. W., Cangir, A., and Taylor, G.: Vincristine sulfate in management of Wilms' tumor. Replacement of preoperative irradiation by chemotherapy. *JAMA* **202**:381–384, 1967.

10. Fernbach, D. J., and Martyn, D. T.: Role of dactinomycin in the improved survival of children with Wilms' tumor. *JAMA* **195**:129–134, 1966.

11. Johnson, D. G., Maceira, F. and Koop, C. E.: Wilms' tumor treated with actinomycin D: the relationship of age and extent of disease to survival. *J. Pediatr. Surg.* **2**:13–27, 1967.

12. Margolis, L. W., Smith, W. B., Wara, W. M., Kushner, J. H., and de Lorimier, A. A.: Wilms' tumor; on interdisciplinary treatment program with and without dactinomycin. *Cancer* **32**:618–622, 1973.

13. Perez, C. A., Kariman, M. A., Keith, J., Mill, W. B., Vietti, T. J., and Powers, W. E.: Treatment of Wilms' tumor and factors affecting prognosis. *Cancer* **32**:609–617, 1973.

14. Burgert, E. O., and Glidewell, O.: Dactinomycin in Wilms' tumor. *JAMA* **199**:124–128, 1967.

15. Wolff, J. A., D'Angio, G., Hartmann, J., Krivit, W., and Newton, W.: Long-term evaluation of single versus multiple courses of actinomycin D therapy of Wilms' tumor. *New Engl. J. Med.* **290**:84–86, 1974.

16. Cassady, J. R., Tefft, M., Filler, R. M., Jaffe, N., Paed, D., and Hellman, S.: Considerations in the radiation therapy of Wilms' tumor. *Cancer* **32**:598–608, 1973.

17. Van Putten, W. J.: Presentation at the British Association of Pediatric Surgeons.

18. Pochedly, C.: Two-and-one-half-year survival of patient with ruptured Wilms' tumor. *JAMA* **216**:334, 1971.

19. Westra, P., Kieffer, S. A., and Mosser, D. G.: Wilms' tumor. A summary of 25 years experience before actinomycin D. *Am. J. Roentgenol.* **100**:214–221, 1967.

20. National Wilms' Tumor Study: Preliminary data supplied courtesy of all the contributors and G. J. D'Angio and J. B. Beckwith, 1975.

21. Woodhead, D. M., Gigax, J. H., Wahle, W. H., and Holcomb, T. M.: Urothelial implantation of Wilms' tumors. *Ann. Surg.* **167**:127–131, 1968.

22. Wang, A. H., Gibbons, I. S. E., Nedwich, A., and Barbero, G. J.: Wilms' tumor associated with venous thrombosis and consumption coagulopathy. *Am. J. Dis. Child.* **123**:599–601, 1972.

23. Vaeth, J. M., and Levitt, S. H.: Five-year results in the treatment of Wilms' tumor of children. *J. Urol.* **90**:247–249, 1963.

24. Scott, L. S.: Wilms' tumor, its treatment and prognosis. *Br. Med. J.* **1**:200–213, 1956.

25. Martin, L. W., and Reyes, P. M.: An evaluation of 10 years with retroperitoneal lymph node dissection for Wilms' tumor. *J. Pediatr. Surg.* **4**:684–687, 1969.

26. Tobin, C. E.: The renal fascia and its relation to the transversalis fascia. *Anat. Rec.* **89**:295–311, 1944.

27. Murphy, D. A., Rabinovitch, H., Chevalier, L., and Virmani, S.: Wilms' tumor in right atrium. *Am. J. Dis. Child.* **126**:210–211, 1973.

28. Sullivan, M. P., Hussey, D. H., and Ayala, A. G.: Wilms' tumor. In: Sutow, W. W., Vietti, T. J., and Fernbach, D. J. (Eds.): *Clinical Pediatric Oncology,* St. Louis, C. V. Mosby Company, 1973, pp. 359–383.

29. Jareb, B.: Metastases and recurrences in nephroblastoma. *Acta Radiol.* **12**:289–303, 1973.

30. Wara, W. M., Margolis, L. W., Smith, W. B., Kushner, J. H., and de Lorimier, A. A.: Treatment of metastatic Wilms' tumor. *Radiology* **112**:695–697, 1974.

31. Monson, K. J., Brand, W. N., and Boggs, J. D.: Results of small-field irradiation of apparent solitary metastasis from Wilms' tumor. *Radiology* **104**:157–160, 1972.

32. Wohl, M. B., Griscom, N. T., Traggis, D. G., and Jaffe, N.: Effects of therapeutic irradiation delivered in early childhood upon subsequent lung function. *Pediatrics* **55**:507–516, 1975.

33. Kilman, J. W., Kronenberg, M. W., D'Neill, J. A., and Klassen, K. P.: Surgical resection for pulmonary metastases in children. *Arch. Surg.* **99**:158–165, 1969.

34. Filler, R. M., Tefft, M., Vawter, G. F., Maddock, C., and Mitus, A.: Hepatic lobectomy in childhood: effects of x-ray and chemotherapy. *J. Pediatr. Surg.* **4**:31–41, 1969.

35. Smith, W. B., Wara, W. M., Margolis, L. W., Kushner, J. H., and de Lorimier, A. A.: Partial hepatectomy in metastatic Wilms' tumor. *J. Pediatr.* **84**:259–261, 1974.

36. Roback, S. A., Nesbit, M. E., Sharp, H. L., D'Angio, G. J., and Leonard, H. S.: Portal hypertension following surgery, x-radiation, and actinomycin D therapy for nephroblastoma. *J. Pediatr.* **78**:1031–1034, 1971.

37. Collins, V. D., Loeffler, R. K., and Tivey, H.: Observations on growth rates of human tumors. *Am. J. Roentgenol.* **76**:988–1000, 1956.

38. Joseph, W. L., Morton, D. L., and Adkins, D. C.: Prognostic significance of tumor doubling time in evaluating operability in pulmonary metastatic disease. *J. Thorac. Cardiovasc. Surg.* **61**:23–31, 1971.

CHAPTER TWELVE

The Role of Radiation Therapy in the Management of Wilms' Tumor

MELVIN TEFFT, M.D.

Attending Radiotherapist
Memorial Hospital for Cancer and Allied Diseases
Professor of Radiology
Cornell University Medical College
New York, New York

CONTENTS

R adiation therapy is used in the management of Wilms' tumor (1) as part of the management of the primary tumor, and (2) as part of the management of metastatic tumor.

RADIATION THERAPY IN MANAGEMENT OF PRIMARY WILMS' TUMOR

The use of irradiation in Wilms' tumor requires knowledge of the clinical extent of the disease in order to determine the volume of tissue to be subtended by the radiation beam. The aim is to include all real and potential tumor-bearing tissue, and to exclude all possible normal tissue from the irradiation beam.

A clinical grouping system (Table 1) devised for the National Wilms' Tumor Study (NWTS) is a method of grouping patients by extent of initial disease and, therefore, is useful to the radiotherapist for alignment of the irradiation beam to the volume to be subtended.[1] The patient's group is decided by the surgeon in the operating room and confirmed by the pathologist. If the histologic diagnosis and grouping will take more than 48 hours, the surgical grouping stands and the patient is registered and started on treatment. If subsequent pathological evaluation leads to regrouping, the fact is reported to the randomization center and the patient is rerandomized for the new Group.

In 1950, Gross and Neuhauser[2] published the results of the treatment of Wilms' tumor at the Children's Hospital Medical Center in Boston. These results describe the survival of children with Wilms' tumor in the years from 1940 through 1947. The survival rate was reported as 47.3%. At that time, this percentage of survival was the highest reported to date and was a significant improvement compared to the survival rates at the Children's Hospital Medical Center during the years 1931 through 1939 (32.2%) and 1914 through 1930 (19%). The authors believed that the unusually high survival of 47.3% from 1940 through 1947, compared to reports from other centers and their own previous experience, was due to the routine use of radiation therapy to the renal fossa of all patients, including those patients who would now be grouped in Group I of the NWTS classification. Since that report, the role of radiation therapy to the renal fossa in Wilms' tumor has become routine at many centers.

Such a portal for irradiation of the renal fossa has encompassed the tissues in which the involved kidney was located and any extension of disease beyond this (Figure 1). The margins of the portal are determined by the original intravenous pyelogram (IVP) and the extent of tumor as determined at surgery. Silver clips placed at the margins of tumor extent at laparotomy will demarcate conveniently the volume for irradiation, as will be apparent on follow-up radiographic examinations. Moreover, any change in position of silver clips on long-term follow-up radiographs of the abdomen could indicate early evidence of local tumor recurrence.

Table 1.   Clinical Grouping According to Criteria of the National Wilms' Tumor Study

GROUP I.   *Tumor limited to kidney and completely resected.* The surface of the renal capsule is intact. The tumor was not ruptured before or during removal. There is no residual tumor apparent beyond the margins of resection.

GROUP II.   *Tumor extends beyond the kidney but is completely resected.* There is local extenstion of the tumor; i.e., penetration beyond the pseudocapsule into the perirenal soft tissues, or periaortic lymph node involvement. The renal vessels outside the kidney substance are infiltrated or contain tumor thrombus. There is no residual tumor apparent beyond the margins of resection.

GROUP III.   *Residual nonhematogenous tumor confined to abdomen.* Any one or more of the following occur: (1) the tumor has been biopsied or ruptured before or during surgery; (2) there are implants on peritoneal surfaces; (3) there are involved lymph nodes beyond the abdominal periaortic chains; or (4) the tumor is not completely resectable because of local infiltration into vital structures.

GROUP IV.   *Hematogenous metastases.* Deposits beyond Group III, e.g., to lung, liver, bone, and brain.

GROUP V.   *Bilateral renal involvement either initially or subsequently.*

The superior extent of the portal for renal fossa irradiation is the superior extent of the involved kidney and mass lesion. In instances where the lesion is large and infiltrative, the superior extent of the portal for irradiation may require the use of the dome of the ipsilateral diaphragm. The inferior border is determined by the lowest extent of the tumor and/or the involved kidney, which is determined by the IVP and/or the findings observed at laparotomy. The lateral border of the portal is described as the lateral abdominal wall with inclusion of the entire peritoneal surface of the ipsilateral renal fossa. The medial border of the irradiation beam subtends both epiphyseal growth centers of the vertebral bodies but does not extend further into the contralateral hemiabdomen. Thus, direct irradiation of the contralateral kidney is avoided. The anterior and posterior opposed portals are utilized in a "weighting" of 1:1 distribution, that is, an equal dose is delivered to the midplane of the renal fossa through the anterior and posterior portals. Ideally, for improved patient tolerance to irradiation, one-half of the planned midplane dose per day should be delivered through each of the two portals on each treatment day. Lateral portals are not utilized since (1) they would deliver direct irradiation to the contralateral kidney through the "exit" beam, and (2) they would deliver an asymmetric dose distribution to the subtended vertebral body.

ANTERIOR PORTAL FOR
RENAL FOSSA IRRADIATION

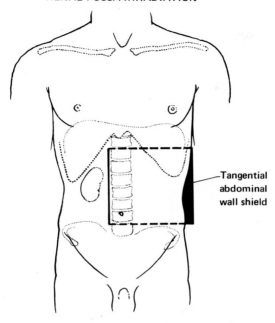

Tangential
abdominal
wall shield

Figure 1. Anterior portal for renal fossa irradiation. The medial border crosses the midline to include both epiphyseal growth centers but does not include direct irradiation of the contralateral kidney. The lateral border includes the entire peritoneal surface of the renal fossa, but a lead shield excludes tangential beam irradiation. The upper and lower borders are determined by the extent of the tumor and its kidney of origin as noted by the IVP and/or laparotomy findings.

Care must be taken to include all the real and potential tumor-bearing tissue while, at the same time, excluding all possible normal tissue from unnecessary irradiation. Thus, the lateral border of the renal fossa portal is tailored in such a way that no tangential beam of irradiation is delivered from the opposed anterior/posterior portals on the lateral skin surface. This is done with external shielding, as indicated in Figure 1. However, the shielding must not be so excessive that any portion of the lateral peritoneal surface is included in the shielded area. As a general rule, shielding the lateral extent of the portal by shielding to within 5 mm of the skin surface obviates the problem of tangential beam irradiation while simultaneously preventing the shielding of peritoneal surfaces. The inferior margin of the portal should exclude all soft tissue and bony tissue of the pelvis unless definite tumor extension into the pelvis is present. If there is evidence of such extension then part or all of the bony and soft tissues of the pelvis must be included in the irradiation beam. Care should be taken to exclude irradiation of the contralateral ovary, and consideration should be given to relocating the contralateral ovary to the soft tissue of the lateral wall of the contralateral pelvis or to the contralateral pelvic brim.[3,4]

The medial border of the portal must subtend both vertebral body growth centers, while not extending into the contralateral hemiabdomen beyond the tip of the contralateral transverse processes mentioned earlier. This allows for symmetric irradiation of vertebral bodies subtended by the beam of irradiation, and excludes the contralateral kidney from the direct beam of irradiation.

The superior margin of the portal should extend above the level of the extent of the renal tumor and the kidney of origin. If, however, the extent of the tumor is either indefinite or diffuse, or if the tumor is invading the hemidiaphragm, then the portal should extend around the dome of the ipsilateral hemidiaphragm. In such instances, care must be taken to exclude cardiac and pulmonary tissue from the direct beam of irradiation by external beam shielding.

Irradiation is delivered at the rate of 150 to 200 rads per day on the basis of a 5-day/wk schedule. The total dose of irradiation should be adjusted to the age of the patient according to the formula shown in Table 2.

When disease is more extensive than that described for Group I and II patients, and when the whole abdomen is at risk in some Group III patients, the portals for irradiation should encompass larger volumes than those described for Group I and II patients. If the residual disease extends beyond the renal fossa the entire abdomen may require irradiation. If there are diffuse peritoneal implants or rupture of the tumor throughout the peritoneal cavity during the surgical procedure, irradiation of the whole abdomen is required. In such instances, the volume subtended for whole abdominal irradiation includes all the peritoneal surfaces, from the tips of the diaphragmatic dome down to and including the entire pelvic contents (Figure 2A, 3). One should, however, exclude the femoral heads from the direct irradiation beam. The remaining kidney should be shielded from the posterior portal, as of the first day of radiation therapy, using four half-value layers

Table 2.   Dosage of Postoperative Radiotherapy for Wilms' Tumor Adjusted to Age of the Patient

Age (months)	Total Tumor Dose (rads)
Birth to 18	1800 to 2400
19 to 30	2400 to 3000
31 to 40	3000 to 3500
41	3500 to 4000

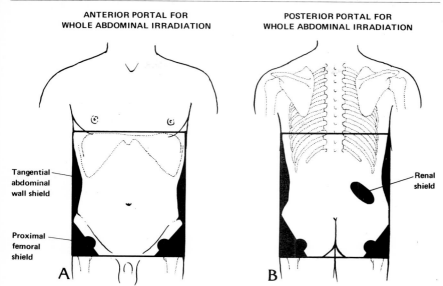

Figure 2.   Portals for whole abdominal irradiation. *(A)* anterior, and *(B)* posterior. The superior margin is at the level of the hemidiaphragm. The inferior margin is at the level of the pubic symphysis, to include all peritoneal tissues of the pelvis. Lead shields are used to exclude tangential beam irradiation and femoral growth centers. A lead shield is also used for the contralateral kidney on the posterior field.

of lead. The daily dose to the midplane of the abdomen should be 150 rads, and 5 treatments delivered per week, for a total dose of 3000 rads to the entire abdominal contents in 4 weeks. Thereafter a higher dose, as described previously for renal fossa irradiation, should be delivered to the region of the renal fossa consistent with the patient's age. For children under 3 years of age, the total dose to the entire abdomen should not exceed 2400 rads in 3 to 3½ weeks.

RADIATION THERAPY IN MANAGEMENT OF METASTATIC WILMS' TUMOR

Lung

Approximately 90% of patients with metastatic disease will demonstrate metastases to the lungs only. Therefore irradiation for metastatic Wilms' tumor entails the need for pulmonary irradiation in most patients who exhibit dissemination.

Irradiation to the lungs for metastatic Wilms' tumor requires irradiating all pulmonary tissue from and including the apices of the lungs to and including the costophrenic sulci at the level of T-12 to L-1. This is done irrespective of the

**ANTERIOR PORTAL FOR BILATERAL
AN PULMONARY IRRADIATION**

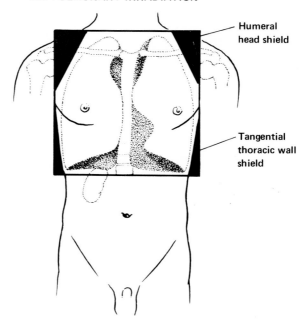

Humeral
head shield

Tangential
thoracic wall
shield

Figure 3.   Portal for bilateral pulmonary irradiation. The fields include shielding of the humeral head and for tangential beam irradiation along the lateral thoracic wall. Both lung fields are included in their entirety, from the level of the pulmonary apices down to and including the costophrenic sulci. The inferior portion of the field is usually at the level of T-12 to L-1.

number of metastases that may be shown on routine chest x-rays. The majority of patients with pulmonary metastases will exhibit more than a solitary metastasis. This being the case, all pulmonary tissue is at risk and must be included in fields of irradiation because of the tendency to "shower."[5] Thus, nonirradiation of any portion of lung in a patient with pulmonary metastases due to Wilms' tumor significantly increases the risk of missing occult metastases. Such nonirradiated lung may later show metastases due to the propensity for showering of micrometastases. Thus underirradiation by volumes less than whole lung irradiation entails a significant risk of overlap of adjacent areas of pulmonary tissue if localized fields are used rather than whole lung irradiation. Therefore, in view of the high proportion of widespread dissemination with gross or microscopic involvement in the lung fields, and of the risk of overirradiation of pulmonary tissues when single lesions are treated through localized irradiation, the concept of whole lung irradiation at initial evidence of pulmonary metastases, irrespective of the numbers of lesions obvious on chest film, has become routine in most centers.

A dose of 1400 rads is delivered in 7 to 10 treatments at the rate of 140 to 200 rads/day, 5 treatments per week. A residual nodule or nodules may be irradiated to a higher dose (a total of 4000 rads in 4 weeks), if no more than 25% of the total volume of both lung fields is subtended in this smaller portal. Repetition of a course of bilateral pulmonary irradiation should be prohibited. Recent review has shown that retrieval is low (about 10%) and morbidity and mortality due to lung fibrosis is high (100%).[5]

Liver

In cases of liver metastases, lesions may be isolated and solitary and may well be amenable to partial hepatic resection. The need for postoperative irradiation depends on the probability of residual disease in the liver. If therapy is to be delivered after partial liver resection, then radiation therapy and/or chemotherapy should not be instituted until full liver regeneration has occurred. This requires approximately 3 to 4 weeks following resection. Liver regeneration is monitored by routine isotopic liver scans performed at weekly intervals. Immediately following partial hepatic resection, one will note an increased radioisotopic distribution in the spleen as compared to the liver and also abnormalities in routine liver function tests. Over the ensuing weeks, reversal of the increased distribution in the enlarged spleen will diminish and the liver function tests will return toward normal. During this time the volume of remaining liver tissue will increase significantly as the liver regenerates. When the plateauing of liver regeneration has occurred, irradiation and/or chemotherapy may begin. The total dose of irradiation to the liver following partial hepatic resection should not exceed 2500 rads in 3 weeks.[6]

In patients who exhibit disease metastatic throughout the liver, and/or in patients who have relatively isolated liver metastasis but who do not undergo partial hepatic resection, the dose to the entire unresected liver should not exceed 3000 rads in 4 weeks. When disease is localized to a portion of the unresected liver, however, the dose may be 4500 rads in 5 weeks. This dose should only be given if no more than two-thirds the volume of the intact liver is subtended by the portal for radiation therapy.

Brain

Disease metastatic to more unusual locations, such as the brain, may require radiation therapy. A recent review[7] showed that in several (approximately 5%) Wilms' tumor patients who exhibited brain metastases, the metastasis have appeared to be solitary in each instance. With effective systemic chemotherapy, a higher percentage of patients may now be retrieved even among those with metastatic disease in the liver and lung. Because of this success aggressive management of metastatic foci in the brain, which might be termed "sanctuary" to routine systemic chemotherapeutic agents, should be the policy.

When the metastatic tumor is in a location suitable for excision, the patient should undergo craniotomy for excision. This should be followed by irradiation to the local tumor bed to a dose of 4000 rads in 4 weeks. Such aggressive management might well permit the long-term survival that has been reported recently.[7]

PREOPERATIVE RADIATION THERAPY

We do not recommend routine use of preoperative irradiation. However, when the primary tumor is so large that even the most experienced surgeon believes there is a significant risk of intraoperative rupture, preoperative radiation therapy may be indicated. In a child who is too ill medically to undergo surgery, and where surgery may be delayed unduly, some form of preoperative therapy to control the local tumor growth would seem indicated. However, in an era of chemotherapy, and with the experience of preoperative administration of vincristine,[8] one must balance morbidities of preoperative therapies. Thus the use of preoperative vincristine would be recommended over that of preoperative irradiation. It should be noted, however, that a recent study by the International Society of Pediatric Oncology has indicated that, in their experience, the routine use of preoperative irradiation has significantly reduced the risk of intraoperative tumor rupture.[9]

DISCUSSION AND COMMENTARY

Adverse Side Effects of Radiation Therapy

By adhering to the guidelines described previously, the degree of radiation effect on normal supporting tissue should be minimized. In 1952, Neuhauser et al.[10] described an increased sensitivity of vertebral body growth and an abnormality of trabecular pattern in children who had received irradiation by portals similar to those described. Since then, the experimental and clinical literature on bone growth abnormality following irradiation has been reviewed.[11] The age-adjusted dose to the renal fossa, as recommended earlier, should result in minimal change of trabecular architecture in the irradiated vertebral body and relatively minimal to moderate disturbance in height.

A minimal degree of scoliosis will occur nonetheless, approximately 12° in the average child. Scoliosis may be due to several factors. There may be fibrosis of the ipsilateral renal fossa and consequent bowing due to contracture secondary to surgery and postoperative irradiation. There may be alteration of vertebral body growth due to disruption of the blood supply to the vertebral body by the presence of the tumor. Penumbra ("fall-off") may occur at the medial edge of the beam, resulting in delivery of a slightly inhomogeneous distribution of radiation to the growth centers of the irradiated vertebral body. Finally, scoliosis may be due to compensatory pelvic tilt in patients who have irradiation of one hemipelvis.[11] A shortening of the sitting height of some degree might be expected, especially if the irradiation is given during the two periods of accelerated growth spurts: ages 1 through 6 years and 11 through 13 years.[12] However, since only a portion of the spine is included in the treatment portal in the postoperative Wilms' tumor patient, the overall degree of shortening should be less than that reported when the entire spine receives irradiation, as in treatment of other clinical conditions.[12]

Physiologic disturbance of normal tissues resulting from irradiation to the lung,[13] liver,[6,15] and kidney,[14] have been reported. With the volume and doses described earlier, such effects should be minimized. Using renal shielding as described, no more than 1500 rads in 4 elapsed weeks should be delivered to the contralateral kidney even when whole abdominal irradiation is employed. This would include direct irradiation from the anterior (unshielded) portal, transmission through the renal shield on the posterior portal, and side scatter to the kidney from surrounding tissues. This dose should be within the limits of renal tolerance.[14]

In a similar fashion, a maximum dose of 3000 rads in 4 weeks to the entire intact liver, with a higher dose of 4500 rads in 5 weeks to the portion of intact liver as described, should not produce evidence of clinical liver dysfunction. Minimizing the dose of irradiation to the liver following partial hepatic resection, and awaiting complete liver regeneration should, likewise, reduce the risk of clinical liver dysfunction.[6]

Irradiation of both lung fields in their entirety, even with concomitant chemotherapy, should result in less than a 10% incidence of radiation pneumonitis if the dose is maintained below the 1500 rad level as outlined previously. Without concomitant chemotherapy, doses of 2000 rads might be considered.[16] However, in the management of Wilms' tumor, the routine use of concomitant chemotherapy for pulmonary irradiation is essential. Although the risk of radiation pneumonitis is low, the possibility of subclinical diffusion defects is distinct.[13] As far as we can determine, such patients remain clinically well despite the pulmonary function abnormality which has been reported.

The etiologic relationship of secondary neoplasia to radiation therapy portals is somewhat unclear since patients with carcinoma have a tendency toward spontaneous occurrence of second neoplasma.[17,18] In our own review,[19] however, most secondary neoplasms occurred in fields of radiation therapy. In view of other evidence which seems to relate the delivery of irradiation to the occurrence of secondary neoplasms,[20,21] radiation therapy may be a significant etiologic factor. The relative frequency of the problem is low and is not outweighed by the use of radiation therapy to achieve long-term survival in a high percentage of patients with Wilms' tumor.

Value of Radiation Therapy in Wilms' Tumor

In 1966 Farber[22] reported an 89% survival of all patients who were referred initially to the Children's Cancer Research Foundation of Boston. Of all patients who showed metastatic disease, 60% were retrieved. This excellent survival was due in part to the role of radiation therapy in those patients in whom radiation therapy was used. Such therapy was given to the renal fossa in patients with localized disease and to the whole abdomen in patients who had disease which would now be classified as Group III. Disease metastatic to lungs was treated by irradiation, as we have described earlier; disease metastatic to liver was treated with combinations of surgical resection and irradiation, or irradiation alone in the manner already mentioned. In addition, all patients received actinomycin D.

Cassady et al.[5] have reported patients who have exhibited recurrence in the abdominal cavity. Such recurrences have been related to insufficient volume and/or dose of irradiation, less than 2500 rads, in patients in whom the grouping would have required, retrospectively, larger volume and higher dose. The authors have also indicated that the retrieval of such patients is poor. Others have also noted the efficacy of radiation therapy.[23,24]

The National Wilms' Tumor Study was designed to evaluate the efficacy of maintenance chemotherapy. It was also designed to evaluate the possibility of omitting radiation therapy in Group I patients, who by definition have no evidence of disease in the renal fossa. The potential usefulness of radiation therapy in achieving long-term survival in patients where it is definitively indicated was recognized. But it was the hope of the National Wilms' Tumor Study Committee that radiation therapy might be excluded, at least in a group of patients who possibly did not require radiation therapy as a routine, and in whom chemotherapy would be used to control hematogenous micrometastases. Concern about the secondary effects of irradiation in the very young child caused this aspect of the study to be added. In a controlled and randomized fashion, Group I patients received either (1) postoperative irradiation to the renal fossa with concomitant maintenance chemotherapy or (2) maintenance chemotherapy, but no postoperative irradiation, to the renal fossa. A preliminary report[25] indicates that there is no significant difference in the overall survival at present between the two groups of patients studied. There is no significant increase of recurrence of tumor in the renal fossa of those patients having had no irradiation compared to those who received radiation therapy.

We do not advise the routine use of radiation therapy to the renal fossa in a patient in the Group I category. If there is any question, however, that the patient may not be a true Group I case but may have some evidence of Group II disease, irradiation should be delivered to the renal fossa as we have outlined earlier. Likewise, all Group III patients should have irradiation either to the renal fossa and/or to whole or parts of the abdomen as indicated by the extension of the disease. All Group IV patients should have irradiation to the abdomen and/or renal fossa as indicated by the extent of local disease and, in addition, should have treatment to areas of metastatic sites as we have described previously.

With a total program of surgery and chemotherapy and the program of radiation therapy we have described, one may expect the survival of children with Wilms' tumor to approach a 100% cure rate, depending on the stage of disease at diagnosis. With proper radiotherapeutic technique, one may expect this with a relatively minimal morbidity from irradiation of the normal soft tissues.

SUMMARY

Radiation therapy has a major role following surgical resection of tumor in patients with a high propensity for residual tumor in the renal fossa, that is, patients in Group II or III. The proper use of radiation therapy in such patients, in terms of dose and volume, should minimize renal fossa recurrence and normal tissue damage.

In patients with disease metastatic to sites such as lung, liver, and brain, the judicious use of radiation therapy allows us to realize a higher percentage of long-term survivors.

In all patients, radiation therapy is combined with concomitant chemotherapy.

REFERENCES

1. Beckwith, B., Breslow, N., Bishop, H., et al.: National Wilms' Tumor Study progress report. Proc. Natl. Cancer Conf. 7: 627–636, 1973.
2. Gross, R. E., and Neuhauser, E. B.: Treatment of mixed tumors of the kidney in childhood. Pediatrics 6: 843–852, 1950.
3. D'Angio, G. J., and Tefft, M.: Radiation therapy in the management of children with gynecological cancers. Ann. N. Y. Acad. Sci. 142: 675–693, 1967.
4. Nisce, L. Z., Geller, W., and D'Angio, G. J.: Experience with a new technique for total nodal irradiation of Hodgkin's disease. Br. J. Radiol. 47: 108–111, 1974.
5. Cassady, J. R., Tefft, M., Filler, R. M., et al.: Considerations in the radiation therapy of Wilms' tumor. Cancer 32: 598–608, 1973.
6. Tefft, M., Mitus, A., Das, L., et al.: Irradiation of the liver in children; review of experience in the acute and chronic phases, and in the intact normal and partially resected. Am. J. Roentgenol. 108: 365–385, 1970.
7. Traggis, D., Jaffe, N., Tefft, M., and Vawter, G.: Successful treatment of Wilms' tumor with intracranial metastases. Pediatrics. In press, 1975.
8. Sullivan, M. P., Sutow, W. W., Cangir, A., and Taylor, G.: Vincristine sulfate in management of Wilms' tumor. JAMA 202: 381–384, 1967.
9. Personal communication, 1974.

10. Neuhauser, E. G., Wittenborg, M. H., Berman, C. Z., and Cohen, J.: Irradiation effects of roentgen therapy on the growing spine. *Radiology* **59**: 637–650, 1952.

11. Tefft, M.: Radiation effect on growing bone and cartilage. *Front. Radiat. Ther. Oncol.* **6**: 289–311, 1972.

12. Probert, J. C., Parker, B. R., and Kaplan, H. S.: Growth retardation in children after megavoltage irradiation of the spine. *Cancer* **32**: 634–639, 1973.

13. Jaffe, N., Wohl, M., Traggis, D. and Griscom, N. T.: Pulmonary function in children treated with pulmonary irradiation (P-XRT) and actinomycin D (AMD) and AMD alone. *Proc. Am. Coll. Radiol.* **14**:124, 1973.

14. Mitus, A., Tefft, M., and Fellers, F. X.: Long-term followup of renal functions of 108 children who underwent nephrectomy for malignant disease. *Pediatrics* **44**: 912–921, 1969.

15. Tefft, M., Traggis, D., and Filler, R. M.: Liver irradiation in children; acute changes with transient leukopenia and thrombocytopenia. *Am. Roentgenol.* **106**: 750–764, 1969.

16. Wara, W. M., Phillips, T. L., Margolis, L. W., and Smith, V.: Radiation pneumonitis; a new approach to the derivation of time-dose factors. *Cancer* **32**: 547–552, 1973.

17. Watson, T. A.: Incidence of multiple cancer. *Cancer* **6**: 365–371, 1953.

18. Moertel, C. G., Dockerty, M. B., and Baggenstoss, A. H.: Multiple primary malignant neoplasms. *Cancer* **14**: 221–248, 1961.

19. Tefft, M., Vawter, G. F., and Mitus, A.: Second primary neoplasms in children. *Am. J. Roentgenol.* **103**: 800–822, 1968.

20. Conard, R. A., Rall, J. E., and Sutow, W. W.: Thyroid nodules as a late sequela of radioactive fallout. *N. Engl. J. Med.* **274**: 1391–1399, 1966.

21. Hempelmann, L. H., Pifer, J. W., Burke, G. J., et al.: Neoplasms in persons treated with x-rays in infancy for thymic enlargement; a report of the third follow-up surgery. *J. Natl. Cancer Inst.* **38**: 317–341, 1967.

22. Farber, S.: Chemotherapy in the treatment of leukemia and Wilms' tumor. *JAMA* **198**: 826–836, 1966.

23. Margolis, L. W., Smith, W. B., Wara, W. W., et al.: Wilms' tumor; an interdisciplinary treatment program with and without dactinomycin. *Cancer* **32**: 618–622, 1973.

24. Aron, B. S.: Wilms' tumor; a clinical study of 81 patients. *Cancer* **33**: 637–646, 1974.

25. Wolff, J.: Advances in the treatment of Wilms' tumor. *Cancer.* In press, 1975.

CHAPTER THIRTEEN

Chemotherapeutic Management of Wilms' Tumor

JAMES A. WOLFF, M.D.

Professor of Pediatrics
College of Physicians and Surgeons
Columbia University
New York, New York
and
Attending Pediatrician
Babies Hospital
The Children's Medical and Surgical Center of New York
New York, New York

Supported in part by U.S. Public Health Service Grants CA 03526, CA 13696, and CA 11722.

CONTENTS

O ver the past 20 years the prognosis in Wilms' tumor has improved progressively, so that today the 2-year survival rate for this formerly highly lethal malignant neoplasm has risen to more than 80%. The improved prognosis has resulted primarily from the introduction during this period of effective chemotherapeutic agents. Prior to the advent of chemotherapy, refinements in surgical and radiotherapy techniques had already brought about some decrease in mortality in this disease. Cure rates from nephrectomy and postoperative radiation for the years 1934 to 1960, are shown in Table 1.

Table 1. Survival in Wilms' Tumors Treated with Nephrectomy and Postoperative Radiotherapy

Author	Years	Number of Cases	Percent Survival
Klapproth[1]	1940–1958	423	26
Lattimer et al.[2]	1934–1956	26	42
Gross[3]	1940–1947	38	47
Westra et al.[4]	1936–1960	46	39

FIRST USE OF CHEMOTHERAPY IN WILMS' TUMOR

The first report of an effective chemical agent for Wilms' tumor was published by Farber and associates in 1965.[5] At approximately the same time, a potentiating interaction between radiation therapy and actinomycin D (Cosmegen) was shown in man[6] and somewhat later experimentally in animals.[7] The enhanced effect of combining actinomycin D with the previously standard treatment of surgery and postoperative radiotherapy in Wilms' tumor was demonstrated clearly by Farber in 1966[8] (Table 2).

The results shown were obtained in those subjects treated from the time of diagnosis at the Children's Cancer Research Foundation. A lesser response rate occurred in other children referred following initiation of treatment at other institutions, indicating the value of coordinated management from the onset of therapy. As shown in Table 2, only 10 of the 47 survivors who had localized disease at diagnosis developed recurrences or metastases. The relapse rate for all patients with localized disease was 30%. Of the children with metastatic disease at diagnosis, 53% survived. A standardized regimen of chemotherapy was not carried out in this study, since some patients received a single course of actinomycin D and others were given maintenance therapy with repeated courses of the drug.

Table 2.   Treatment of Wilms' Tumor with Actinomycin D—Children's Cancer Research Foundation, 1957–1964

	Results of Therapy	
Initial Clinical Status	Alive and Well	Dead
No metastases at onset of therapy		
Without subsequent relapse	37/53	6/53
Following relapse	10/53	
Metastases at onset of therapy	8/15	7/15
All patients	55/68	13/68

USE OF MAINTENANCE CHEMOTHERAPY

At this time it seemed plausible that maintenance actinomycin D treatment might be effective in eradicating possible microscopic metastatic foci in patients with apparent localized disease. Therefore, Children's Cancer Study Group A initiated a randomized clinical trial in 1964 comparing standard treatment with surgery and postoperative radiotherapy plus a single course of actinomycin D at diagnosis to similar standard therapy plus repeated courses of this drug for a 15-month period. The protocol is shown in Table 3. Preliminary evaluation in 1968[9] reported a 52% (12/23) relapse rate in the single course group and 14% (3/22) in those given maintenance actinomycin D; this difference was statistically significant. Subsequent follow-up, reported in 1974,[10] showed a less marked difference in the relapse rates between the two groups, although the difference remained significant on statistical analysis. In 1974 the relapse rate was 57% (16/28) in the single-course group and 28% (7/25) in the maintenance actinomycin D subjects. The relapse rates are shown in Table 4. A greater percentage of relapsed subjects in the single-course actinomycin D group was rescued by subsequent treatment than in the maintenance therapy group. The difference in survival in 1974, 71% versus 80%, was not significant at the 5% level (Table 5).

Multiple courses of drug therapy in this study were primarily effective in suppressing pulmonary metastases, as evidenced by 12 of 16 relapses in the lung alone in the first group and only 1 of 7 in the lung alone in the second (Table 6). The conclusion drawn from the study was that the occurrence of fewer relapses in patients given maintenance actinomycin D, requiring fewer control measures such as additional radiotherapy, administration of other drugs, or surgical excision of recurrent tumors, results in a lower morbidity from the disease and its treatment.

Table 3. Treatment Protocol of Children's Cancer Study Group A: Single-Course Therapy vs. Maintenance Therapy

	Single-Course Therapy	Maintenance Therapy
At diagnosis		
	Surgery Radiotherapy Actinomycin D	Surgery Radiotherapy Actinomycin D
Subsequently		
	No therapy	Actinomycin D at 6 weeks, 3 months, and every 3 months thereafter until 15 months after surgery

Table 4. Relapse Rates of Children's Cancer Study Group A

Type of Chemotherapy	Relapse Rates	
	1968	1974
Single course of actinomycin D	52%	57%
Maintenance of actinomycin D	14%	28%

Table 5. Survival Rate Comparing Single-Course and Maintenance Actinomycin D, Children's Cancer Study Group A, 1974

Type of Chemotherapy	Survival Rate (%)
Single course of actinomycin D	71 (20/28)
Maintenance of actinomycin D	80 (20/25)

USE OF VINCRISTINE

Other chemotherapeutic agents have undergone clinical trial in the treatment of Wilms' tumor. Vincristine (Oncovin) became available for clinical trials in human leukemias and solid tumors in 1962. As reported by Sutow[11] in 1965, this drug was shown to be remarkably effective against Wilms' tumor. Sullivan and Sutow in 1969 reported an 83% disease-free interval with a median of 4½ years in localized Wilms' tumor,[12] and Vietti and associates described a 45% 2-year

Table 6.   Sites of First Relapses, Children's Cancer Study Group A

	Type of Chemotherapy	
Site(s) of First Relapse	Single Course of Actinomycin D	Maintenance of Actinomycin D
Lung only	12	1
Lung and contralateral kidney	0	1
Lung and abdomen	1	0
Mediastinum	1	1
Liver only	2	1
Liver and abdomen	0	1
Bone	0	2
Total	16	7

survival in children with metastatic disease[13] (Table 7). Sullivan et al.[14] have also demonstrated marked shrinkage of massive Wilms' tumors with two weekly preoperative doses of vincristine, allowing relatively easy removal of presumably inoperable primary tumors. The activity of vincristine appeared to parallel the cytotoxic effect of actinomycin D against Wilms' tumor. Both of these drugs also showed greater activity than a number of other chemical agents submitted to clinical trials during the period from 1960 to 1970.

Despite numerous side effects neither actinomycin D nor vincristine, when used as single chemotherapeutic compounds, produce intolerable toxicity. Actinomycin D is not only therapeutically synergistic with radiotherapy but also potentiates its toxicity. Augmentation of radiation-induced toxicity to the skin or soft tissues occurs with its concomitant use, and reactivation of such effects may result from subsequent administration of this agent. Mucositis and bone marrow depression are also encountered. These occur most frequently several days after completion of a 5-day course of treatment. Reversible alopecia occurs in many subjects, especially when repeated courses of the drug are given. Peripheral

Table 7.   Results of Treatment of Wilms' Tumor with Vincristine

Extent of Disease	Disease-free Survival (%)	Follow-up (years)
Localized	83	4½ (median)
Metastatic	45	2

neuropathy is the principal side effect of vincristine. Various manifestations of neural toxicity include pain in the jaw, pain on swallowing, loss of deep tendon reflexes, slapping gait, constipation, and paralytic ileus. Transient fever and an inappropriate ADH syndrome occur occasionally.

Vincristine does not cause significant bone marrow depression, but ineffective erythropoiesis or thrombocytosis may result from its administration. It produces reversible alopecia more frequently than actinomycin D. Both actinomycin D and vincristine must be administered with great care because extravasation of either drug into the tissue surrounding the vein leads to severe chemical irritation. Although apprehension concerning later mutational effects is certainly justified, especially for actinomycin D which binds DNA and inhibits transcription of RNA, to date no late toxicity has been reported for either drug. Both actinomycin D and vincristine are administered intravenously, usually by slow push. The usual dose for a single course of actinomycin D is 0.075 mg/kg given in 5 divided daily doses. The maximum total single dose in 0.5 mg. Vincristine is more frequently given at weekly intervals, in a dose of 1.5 to 2.0 mg/m,[2] not exceeding 2.0 mg for a single dose. For infants, in whom the surface area is relatively large in comparison to weight, both drugs are best calculated on a per kilogram basis in order to avoid undue toxicity.

Despite the improvement in survival from treatment with actinomycin D or vincristine, a number of important questions concerning the treatment of Wilms' tumor were apparent in 1969 and remained to be answered. These included the relative activities of actinomycin D and vincristine, the possible enhanced effect of the two drugs used in combination, the necessity of The annual incidence of newly diagnosed cases of Wilms' tumor in the United States has been estimated by Miller[15] to be approximately 500.

ORIGIN OF THE NATIONAL WILMS' TUMOR STUDY GROUP

The annual incidence of newly diagnosed cases of Wilms' tumor in the United States has been estimated by Miller[15] to be approximately 500. Since the disease was relatively rare, it became evident that answers to the above and other pertinent questions would require many years of randomized trials by individual institutions or even by national cooperative groups. Therefore various groups of specialists concerned with pediatric oncology joined forces in an effort to consolidate their cases, in order to increase the number of patients who could be entered in future clinical trials. The result of these discussions was the creation of the National Wilms' Tumor Study Group in the same year.[16] This Committee represents three of the major national cooperative chemotherapy groups: Children's Cancer Study Group A, Acute Leukemia Group B, and the Southwest Oncology Group, as well as a number of independent investigators.

The first consideration of the newly formed committee was the elaboration of a provisional staging classification for Wilms' tumor that could be utilized for future clinical trials. The following classification was proposed:

Group I—Tumor limited to kidney and completely resected.
Group II—Tumor extends beyond the kidney but is completely resected.
Group III—Residual nonhematogenous tumor confined to abdomen.
Group IV—Hematogenous metastases.
Group V—Bilateral renal involvement.

A National Wilms' Tumor Study was begun on October 1, 1969, to answer the questions noted previously. Table 8 shows the randomization in the various groups of the provisional staging classification.

In Group I all patients were given maintenance therapy with actinomycin D for a period of 15 months. Randomization consisted of the addition of postoperative radiotherapy to patients in regimen A. In staging Groups II and III, all children were treated with postoperative radiotherapy following surgery. In these staging groups, randomization to either one drug alone or to a combination of both drugs for a 15-month treatment period was carried out. Patients in staging Group IV were randomized to preoperative vincristine or no vincristine preoperatively. Actinomycin D in all four groups was given in 5-day courses, 0.015 mg/kg/day, intravenously, at the time of diagnosis, at 6 weeks and 3 months postoperatively, and then every 3 months thereafter for a total period of 15 months. In Groups II and III vincristine was given weekly intravenously 1.5 mg/m^2 for 8 doses beginning at surgery. Subsequently, it was administered on the first and fifth day of the month every 3 months, from 3 months until 15 months after diagnosis. In regimen A of Group IV, vincristine therapy was identical to that in Groups II and III. In regimen B of Group IV, two preoperative doses of vincristine were given at weekly intervals. Patients with Group V disease were registered and followed but not randomized into the study.

From October 1, 1969, to June 30, 1973, 510 subjects were registered. Of these, 82 were not eligible for study because of prior chemotherapy, patient or doctor refusal, or other reasons. Of the total, 308 patients have been randomized; the other 120 subjects are not in the study for various reasons. Of the 120 excluded from the study, 27 had bilateral tumors at diagnosis and 26 had incorrect preoperative diagnoses. Of the nonrandomized subjects, 9 had a histologic diagnosis of mesoblastic nephroma. Prior experience indicated that simple removal of this type of tumor is curative and that radiotherapy and chemotherapy might impose unnecessary morbidity or mortality for such patients. Patient entry in the various randomized staging groups was as follows: Group I, 43%; Group II, 27%; Group III, 21%; and Group IV, 9%.

Table 8. National Wilms' Tumor Study Protocol: Randomization by Staging and Treatment Groups

Staging	Treatment
Group I	R a n d o m i z e Regimen A. SUR* + RT* + AMD* Regimen B. SUR + AMD (no RT)
Groups II and III	R a n d o m i z e Regimen A. SUR + RT + AMD Regimen B. SUR + RT + VCR* Regimen C. SUR + RT + AMD + VCR
Group IV	R a n d o m i z e Regimen A. SUR + RT + AMD + VCR Regimen B. Preop VCR + SUR + RT + AMD + VCR

*Key: SUR = surgery, RT = radiotherapy, AMD = actinomycin D, VCR = vincristine.

Serious toxicity has not been encountered regularly with any of the treatment regimens. Early in the study an increased morbidity was observed in patients receiving combined actinomycin D and vincristine. More recently, presumably as experience has been gained, increased toxicity associated with combined chemotherapy has not been noted.

RESULTS OF THE NATIONAL WILMS' TUMOR STUDY

Preliminary results of this study were reported in 1974.[17] Although definitive conclusions concerning the response to therapy could not be made from the evaluation of all cases through June 30, 1973, because of insufficient numbers of patients, some tentative results emerged. These are shown in Tables 9 and 10. In Group I only one flank relapse had occurred, a patient in the no-radiotherapy randomized arm. The 2-year actuarial disease-free rate in both regimens A and B of Group I, a total of 83 patients, has been equally good and better than 80%. The 2-year actuarial disease-free rates for 94 randomized cases in the combined Groups II and III was 79% for combined actinomycin D and vincristine as compared to 50% for actinomycin D alone and 44% for vincristine alone. The 2-year actuarial survival rate for Group I was 98% for patients given radiotherapy and 95% for those not given radiotherapy. In Groups II and III combined, the 2-year actuarial survival rate was 50% for those given actinomycin D alone, 62% for vincristine alone and 92% for subjects given combined drugs. In 19 patients with hepatic or extraabdominal metastases (Group IV), the use of preoperative vincristine did not show an advantage in this small sample.

Further analysis of the response of patients entered into the National Wilms' Tumor Study through January 31, 1974, currently in progress, does not appear to show differences from the results shown above. Addition of postoperative radiotherapy in Staging Group I patients has not conferred an advantage. The use of two drugs rather than one has continued to produce better responses in Groups II and III. Therefore these trials have been concluded, so that new questions concerning treatment of Wilms' tumor may be investigated in order to improve further the current excellent response rates.

Table 9. Two-Year Actuarial Disease-free Rate, National Wilms' Tumor Study, June 30, 1973

Staging and Therapy	2-Year Disease-free Rate (%)
Group I	
Radiotherapy	> 80
No radiotherapy	
Groups II and III combined	
Actinomycin D alone	50
Vincristine alone	44
Actinomycin D and vincristine	79

Table 10.   Two-Year Actuarial Survival Rate, National Wilms' Tumor Study, June 30, 1973

Staging and Therapy	2-Year Survival Rate (%)
Group I	
Radiotherapy	98
No radiotherapy	95
Groups II and III combined	
Actinomycin D alone	50
Vincristine alone	62
Actinomycin D and vincristine	92

PROSPECTS FOR FUTURE STUDIES

Experience with adriamycin in the treatment of Wilms' tumor has accumulated in the last several years with encouraging results.[18,19] To date, response to treatment of Wilms' tumor with adriamycin has been reported by eight groups of investigators in 51 patients.[20] Of these, 32 (63%) showed some response and 9 (18%) have had complete responses. Therefore the possibility of an even better response rate with a 3-drug regimen, adding adriamycin to vincristine and actinomycin D, should be explored in more advanced disease. The need for a long period (e.g., 15 months) of maintenance drug therapy compared to one of shorter duraton also deserves consideration in Group I patients. To answer some of these new questions, investigations on a national level would be desirable.

The National Wilms' Tumor Study Committee will conduct randomized trials in the near future to compare response rates in Group I patients treated following nephrectomy with combined actinomycin D and vincristine without postoperative radiotherapy for a 6-month period compared to a 15-month period. For Groups II, III, and IV patients, comparison of a 2-drug regimen (actinomycin D and vincristine) with a 3-drug regimen (actinomycin D, vincristine, and adriamycin) in addition to surgery and radiotherapy will be evaluated.

SUMMARY

The addition in the past 20 years of chemotherapy to other treatment modalities for Wilms' tumor has resulted in greatly improved survival in this formerly highly lethal malignant neoplasm of childhood. Although actinomycin D and vincristine are each effective therapeutic agents, their combined use has produced an even greater improvement in outlook. Thus far recent studies have not shown an advantage in patients with localized, completely resected tumors from the use of postoperative radiotherapy. Future investigations will assess the value of the addition of another effective compound, adriamycin, in more advanced disease.

REFERENCES

1. Klapproth, H. J.: Wilms' tumor; a report of 45 cases and an analysis of 1,351 cases reported in the world literature from 1940 to 1950. *J. Urol.* 81: 633, 1959.

2. Lattimer, J. K., Melicow, M. M., and Uson, A. C.: Wilms' tumor; a report of 71 cases. *J. Urol.* 80: 401, 1958.

3. Gross, R. E., *The Surgery of Infancy and Childhood*, W. B. Saunders Company, Philadelphia, 1953, p 602.

4. Westra, P., Kieffer, S. A., and Mosser, D. G.: Wilms' tumor; a summary of 25 years of experience before actinomycin D. *Am. J. Roentgenol.* 100: 214, 1967.

5. Farber, S., Toch, R., Sears, E. M., and Pinkel, D.: Advances in chemotherapy of cancer in man. In *Advances in Cancer Research*, Vol. IV, Academic Press, New York, 1956, pp. 1–71.

6. D'Angio, G. J., Farber, S., and Maddock, C. L.: Potentiation of x-ray effects by actinomycin D. *Radiology* 73: 197, 1959.

7. D'Angio, G. J., Maddock, C. L., Farber, S., and Brown, B. L.: Enhanced response of Ridgeway osteogenic sarcoma to roentgen radiation combined with actinomycin D. *Cancer Res.* 25: 1003, 1965.

8. Farber, S.: Chemotherapy in the treatment of leukemia and Wilms' tumor. *JAMA* 108: 826, 1966.

9. Wolff, J. A., Krivit, W., Newton, W. A., Jr., and D'Angio, G. J.: Single versus multiple dose dactinomycin therapy of Wilms' tumor; controlled cooperative study conducted by the Children's Cancer Study Group A. *N. Engl. J. Med.* 279: 290, 1968.

10. Wolff, J. A., D'Angio, G. J., Hartmann, J., et al.: Long-term evaluation of single versus multiple courses of actinomycin D therapy of Wilms' tumor. *N. Engl. J. Med.* 290: 84, 1974.

11. Sutow, W. W.: Chemotherapy in childhood cancer; an appraisal. *Cancer* 18: 1585, 1965.

12. Sullivan, M. P., and Sutow, W. W.: Successful therapy for Wilms' tumor. *Texas Med.* 65: 46, 1969.

13. Vietti, T. J., Sullivan, M. P., Haggard, M. E., et al.: Vincristine sulfate and radiation therapy in metastatic Wilms' tumor. *Cancer* 25: 12, 1970.

14. Sullivan, M. P., Sutow, W. W., Cangir, A., and Taylor, G.: Vincristine sulfate in management of Wilms' tumor. *JAMA* 202:38, 1967.

15. Miller, R. W.: Deaths from childhood cancer in siblings. *N. Engl. J. Med.* 279: 122, 1968.

16. D'Angio, G. J., Beckwith, J. B., Bishop, H. C., et al.: The National Wilms' Tumor Study; progress report. *Seventh Natl. Cancer Conf. Proc.* 15: 627, 1973.

17. D'Angio, G. J., Beckwith, J. R., Bishop, H., et al.: The National Wilms' Tumor Study; preliminary results. (abstr.) *Proc. Am. Assoc. Cancer Res., 65th Ann. Meet.*, 1974.

18. Wollner, N., Tan, C., Ghavimi, F., et al.: Adriamycin in childhood leukemia and solid tumors. *Proc. Amer. Assoc. Cancer Res.* 12: 75, 1971 (abstr.)

19. Wang, J. J., Cortes, E., Sinks, L. F., and Holland, J. F.: Therapeutic effect and toxicity of adriamycin in patients with neoplastic disease. *Cancer* 28: 837, 1971.

20. Gottlieb, J.: Personal communication, 1974.

CHAPTER FOURTEEN

Estimating the Prognosis in Wilms' Tumor

D. W. O'GORMAN HUGHES, M.D., M.B., B.S.

Chairman, Division of Pediatric Haematology and Oncology
The Prince of Wales Hospital
Senior Lecturer in Pediatrics
University of New South Wales
Sydney, N.S.W., Australia

CONTENTS

W ilms' tumor is of particular interest to the pediatrician and oncologist for two major reasons. First, of all the childhood malignancies it has the greatest potential for cure even when metastases are present; second, its management exemplifies the importance of the combined roles of surgery, radiotherapy, and chemotherapy. While advances in treatment over the past decade have further improved the survival rate, it is also appropriate to analyze other features at diagnosis that may be of prognositc importance. These features include clinical staging, pathology of the tumor, and age of the patient.

CLINICAL STAGING

Although the findings of completely resectable tumor, local spread, or distant metastases have long been recognized to influence the long-term prognosis, the lack of a uniform and precise clinical staging has seriously hampered the comparison of data between different institutions. The classification by Garcia et al.[1] placed emphasis on the size of the tumor, and cases of unresectable local tumor were not segregated from those with metastases. Fleming and Pinkel[2] and Fleming and Johnson[3] emphasized the necessity for careful staging in correlation with prognosis and treatment, and categorized the disease into four stages. The more recent and widely accepted staging (grouping) by the National Wilms' Tumor Study (NWTS)[4] differs from that of Fleming and Johnson by transferring cases with hepatic involvement into Stage IV and cases of Bilateral Wilms' tumor into a new Stage V.

In Table 1 the proportion of patients surviving beyond 2 years in several series is recorded according to the stages of the disease. Where possible, the stages (groups) were reclassified into the NWTS categories. In some reports complete categorization was not possible, and Stages III to V were grouped together. Even allowing for variations in treatment in different areas a fairly consistent pattern was observed: the proportion of survivors was very high for Stage I patients, good for those with Stage II disease, and much worse for patients with more advanced stages of the disease. The influence of chemotherapy on survival of patients with bilateral Wilms' tumor and metastatic disease is also shown in Table 1, and will be discussed subsequently.

PATHOLOGIC FEATURES

Several reports[7,10,11] have indicated that tumors with a preponderance of epithelial elements and well-formed glomeruloid structures and tubules have less tendency to metastasize and have a better prognosis than tumors with predominantly undifferentiated spindle elements. Currie et al.[5] observed an excellent correlation

217

Table 1. Survival in Wilms' Tumor in Relation to Clinical Staging [a]

Reference	Period	Therapy	Stage (Group)					Total
			I	II	III	IV	V	
Currie et al. (1973)[5]	1956–1969	Nx, RT, AMD	6/10	2/4	1/4		1/3	10/21
Fleming et al. (1970)[3] Survival	1962–1969	Nx, RT, AMD	11/11	3/7	4/12	0/2		18/32
Margolis et al. (1973)[6] Survival, NED	1962–1970	Nx, RT, AMD ± VCR	4/4	8/8	2/2	1/4	3/4	18/22
Perez et al. (1973)[7] Survival, NED	1962–1969	Nx, RT, AMD, VCR	7/7	5/6	0/1	3/7	3/3	18/24
Subtotal[3,5,6,7]		Nx, RT, AMD ± VCR	28/32	18/25	7/19	4/13	7/10	64/99

Reference	Years	Treatment						Total
Margolis et al. (1973)[6] Survival, NED	1945–1961	Nx, RT	8/12	2/3	0/2	0/1	0/3	10/21
Perez et al[7] Survival, NED	1959–1961	Nx, RT	5/8	0/3	0/8	0/3	0/3	5/25
Subtotal[6,7]		Nx, RT	13/20	2/6	0/10	0/4	0/6	15/46
Total[3,5,6,7]	1945–1970	Nx, RT, ± AMD, ± VCR	41/52 (79%)	20/31 (65%)	7/29 (24%)	4/17 (24%)	7/16 (44%)	79/145 (54%)
Cassady et al.[8] (1973)[8]	1960–1970	Nx, RT + AMD ± VCR	11/11	40/48	17/34 --------→			68/93
Maier et al.[9] (1967)[9]	1949–1959	Nx, RT	3/3	8/8	2/13 --------→			13/24
	1960–1965	Nx, RT, AMD	1/1	1/2	3/14 --------→			5/17
Total[3,5–9]	1945–1970		56/67 (84%)	69/89 (78%)	40/123 (32%)			165/279 (59%)

[a] Staging transferred to classification of National Wilms' Tumor Study where possible. Abbreviations: NED no evidence of disease; Nx nephrectomy; RT radiotherapy; AMD actinomycin D: VCR vincristine.

[b] Grouped separately because of difficulties in assessing precise classifications into stages II to V.

219

between the histologic type and prognosis in 21 patients treated between 1956 and 1969 with nephrectomy, postoperative radiotherapy, and actinomycin D. They described three histologic types. In type 1, with abundant tubular elements and well-organized glomerule, epithelial elements comprised > 20% of the areas examined. In type 2 lesions, malignant embryonic stroma predominated but there was some tubular and glomerular formation, with epithelial elements comprising > 5% but < 20% of the tissue observed microscopically. Type 3 lesions were frankly anaplastic and composed almost entirely of embryonic stroma; tubular and glomerular formation was virtually absent and comprised < 5% of the histological fields. All of Currie's 5 type 1 patients survived and 4 of 6 type 2 patients survived, but only 1 of 10 patients with type 3 histology was alive.

Bannayan et al.[12] observed a greater degree of nonepithelial differentiation in metastases as compared to the primary tumors, and suggested that irradiation accelerated and possibly induced the differentiation.

In infancy a benign, congenital mesoblastic nephroma or fetal hamartoma of the kidney was described by Bolande et al.[13] in a series of 8 infants. It was established that this tumor was benign and that nephrectomy was curative. This tumor, frequently misdiagnosed as congenital Wilms' tumor in the past, has undoubtedly contributed to the reported high cure rates of Wilms' tumor in infancy. In a number of major institutions the only neonatal or congenital renal tumors were congenital mesoblastic nephromas.[13-16] It has even been suggested that a malignant Wilms' tumor at birth either does not exist or is extremely rare.[15]

Garcia et al.[1] found a better prognosis in patients whose primary tumor was less than 550 ml. However, in other reports,[7,8] there was no clear correlation between the volume of the neoplasm and survival.

AGE AND PROGNOSIS

The more favorable prognosis in infants with Wilms' tumor has been stated repeatedly over the past 20 years (Table 2), although there was no obvious preference for the younger age groups in some reports.[3,5,8] The better outlook for younger children could be explained partly by the failure to exclude congenital mesoblastic nephromas and by a more favorable staging of the disease in infancy.

In Table 3 an assessment of the age of the patient is compared with the proportion of survivors in three recent reports. These series were selected because extrapolation to the staging classification by the NWTS was possible, the age of demarcation for younger and older children at 2 years was uniform, and the periods of analysis were generally comparable. In the younger age groups nearly 50% of the patients had Stage I disease compared with 25% in the older age group. There was a better outlook for younger patients with Stage I disease, and the difference in prognosis between the two age groups in patients with later stages of the disease was less obvious.

Table 2.   Wilms' Tumor: Age at Diagnosis Compared with Survival

Reference	Period of Study	Age of Demarcation	Survival	
			Younger Children	Older Children
Gross (1953)[17]	1940–1947	12 mo	80%	43%
Scott (1956)[18]	to 1954	12 mo	18% (3/17)	7% (3/46)
Sukarochana and Kiesewetter (1966)[19]	1949–1962	2 yr	51% (18/35)	33% (9/27)
Maier and Harshaw (1967)[9]	1949–1965	2 yr	75% (9/12)	31% (9/29)
Margolis et al. (1973)[6]	1945–1970	2 yr	73% (22/30)	45% (14/33)
Perez et al. (1973)[7]	1950–1969	2 yr	63% (12/19)	37% (11/30)
Currie et al. (1973)[5]	1956–1969	2 yr	50% (5/10)	45% (5/11)
Cassady et al. (1973)[8]	1960–1970	18 mo	83% (15/18)	73% (53/73)
Fleming and Johnson (1970)[3]	1962–1967	2 yr	36% (4/11)	67% (14/21)

Table 3.   Wilms' Tumor: Proportion of Survivors Compared with Age of the Patient and Stage of the Disease

Stage*	I	II	III	IV	V	Total
Age < 2 Years						
Margolis et al. (1973)[6]	11/12	7/7	2/3	—	2/8	22/30
Perez et al. (1973)[7]	10/10	0/3	0/1	0/2	2/3	12/19
Currie et al. (1973)[5]	2/5	2/3	—	—	1/2	5/10
Total	23/27	9/13	2/4	0/2	5/13	39/59
	(85%)	(69%)	(50%)		(38%)	(66%)
Age > 2 Years						
Margolis et al. (1973)[6]	3/8	3/4	6/10	1/6	1/3	14/31
Perez et al. (1973)[7]	2/5	5/6	0/8	3/8	1/3	11/30
Currie et al. (1973)[5]	4/5	0/1	1/4	—	0/1	5/11
Total	9/18	8/11	7/22	4/14	2/7	30/72
	(50%)	(73%)	(32%)	(29%)	(29%)	(42%)

*Staging according to the classification of the National Wilms' Tumor Study.

THE INFLUENCE OF TREATMENT ON SURVIVAL

Surgical excision of the tumor is of major importance in initial management. In a large series reported by Ledlie et al.,[20] no patient treated without nephrectomy survived. The effective role of combining surgery and postoperative radiotherapy was well documented by Gross in Boston. In 1953 he reported the results of treatment in 96 children with Wilms' tumor between 1914 and 1947.[17] During the first period, 1914 to 1930, surgery was performed but adequate supportive measures were not available, and the cure rate was 15%. From 1931 to 1939, when surgery was employed with adequate supportive measures, the cure rate was 32%. In the third period, 1940 to 1947, when surgery was followed by postoperative radiotherapy, the cure rate rose to 47%, being 80% in infants under the age of 1 year and 43% for older children.

The first report of the use of chemotherapy with actinomycin D was by Farber and his co-workers in 1956.[21] Ten years later he summarized the results over a 7-year period.[22] Sixty-eight children with Wilms' tumor received all treatment at the Children's Hospital Medical Center, Boston, and were treated with the combination of nephrectomy, local radiotherapy, and actinomycin D. Of these patients, 53 presented without metastases, 37 had no evidence of subsequent disease at any time, and 10 of 16 who developed subsequent metastases were alive without evidence of disease for at least 2 years following therapy. The 2-year survival rate for this group was 89%. Of 15 additional patients with metastases at diagnosis, 8 (53%) were free of disease 2 to 9 years later. The overall survival rate for the 68 children was 81%. Reports by Howard,[23] Colebatch et al.,[24] and Fernbach and Martyn[25] indicated a greatly improved cure rate when actinomycin D was added to the regimen of surgery and radiotherapy.

In 1968, in a short-term study,[26] the Children's Cancer Study Group A demonstrated the superiority of multiple over single courses of actinomycin D in preventing metastases. The patients, all over the age of 12 months, had localized resectable unilateral tumors (now Stages I and II, NWTS classification). The standard treatment for all surgical resection, a course of actinomycin D (dosage 0.015 mg/kg on 5 successive days), and postoperative irradiation to the tumor bed. Thereafter, one group received similar courses of actinomycin D at 6 weeks and at 3,6,9,12, and 15 months after operation, while the other group received no further chemotherapy. Of 22 children given multiple course, 19 (86%) had no recurrence compared with 11 of 23 (48%) given a single course. In a subsequent report,[27] with a minimum follow-up period of 4 years, the relapse rate was still lower in the multiple course group (7 of 25, 28%) than in the single course group (16 of 28, 57%). Metastases to the lungs were the most frequent site of relapse in the single course group, but rarely occurred after multiple courses. It was concluded that actinomycin D at repeated intervals was highly effective in preventing most pulmonary metastases. However, the overall survival in the two groups was similar (80% vs. 70%) as a higher proportion of the relapsing patients in the single course group subsequently survived.

Vincristine has also proved a potent chemotherapeutic agent in Wilms' tumor. Significant regression in 8 of 12 patients with metastases was reported by the Southwest Cancer Chemotherapy Group in 1963, but the response was short-lived.[28] In 1970 the same group reported complete regression of metastatic disease in 16 of 22 children treated with vincristine and radiation to the metastases.[30] Of the children, 10 (45%) were alive and free of obvious disease for more than 2 years after treatment of their metastases, and the survival figures might have improved if radiotherapy had been given to all metastatic sites.

The optimum treatment for Wilms' tumor has yet to be completely defined, and studies in progress by the National Wilms' Tumor Study[4] may answer some questions. Preliminary results suggest that radiotherapy to the tumor bed in Stage I disease may offer no additional benefits of the combination of surgery and chemotherapy.[4] The relative merits of actinomycin D and vincristine are not yet clearly delineated, although both are effective chemotherapeutic agents whether used singly or in combination. Given optimal clinical circumstances, it has been suggested from calculations that long-term survival when both actinomycin D and vincristine are used could exceed 90% in nonmetastatic disease and 60% in patients with metastases.[29,39]

Metastatic disease, especially that involving the lungs, has usually been treated with actinomycin D with or without vincristine and radiotherapy. There is good evidence that radiation therapy alone is far less effective than radiotherapy with actinomycin D for metastatic disease.[30] The salvage rate using mainly actinomycin D and radiation therapy has usually been 40 to 50%, with extremes of 30 to 100% in small series,[7,8,21,22] Vietti et al.[30] reported 45% disease-free survival employing vincristine and radiation to metastases; at further follow-up of 5 patients treated similarly by O'Gorman Hughes et al.,[32] 4 remained free of disease off treatment at 2½ years. Recurrence developed in 1 patient, but after resection of a solitary metastasis and chemotherapy she is again disease-free.

Evidence has been presented that multiple pulmonary metastases or widespread dissemination to other organs are less likely to respond to chemotherapy and radiation.[8,40] Cassady et al.[8] observed that with two exceptions, only the patients who relapsed with pulmonary metastases alone could be salvaged by subsequent aggressive therapy. Local recurrences, which rarely occur with Stage I disease, have been observed mainly in children with evidence of metastatic disease[7,8] and are usually of sinister prognostic import.

Other measures that have improved the survival rate with massive primary tumors are preoperative chemotherapy and local radiotherapy.[33,34] Waggett and Koop described the use of these modalities in management of 12 cases of massive Wilms' tumor.[33] All 5 patients without metastases and 4 of 7 with metastases were alive and free of disease. Surgical resection of metastases, which may be combined with chemotherapy and radiotherapy, has also been utilized with good results in selected cases.[31,35]

The outlook for bilateral Wilms' tumor is not as hopeless as may have been anticipated. In five series, 16 of 26 patients were alive without evidence of disease; in a review of the literature Ragab et al. reported that 40% of 70 patients were considered cured.[36] Judicious surgery combined with radiotherapy and chemotherapy have been responsible for these remarkable results.

ASSESSMENT OF THE OVERALL PROGNOSIS

Collins devised the concept of a period of risk for recurrence.[37] If the patient survived for a period exceeding his age at diagnosis plus 9 months a cure was likely. Although this period of risk is a useful measurement it has the disadvantage of prolonged waiting to assess results. Cassady et al. found that 4% of their patients suffered relapse beyond the duration of Collins' period of risk.[8] A more rapid and useful measurement is the estimation of the status of the patient 2 years from diagnosis. If there is no evidence of recurrence, there are prospects for cure in more than 90% of patients.[6,8] The modern combinations of treatment may suppress the clinical manifestations of recurrence until some time after the cessation of chemotherapy, and further risk periods may need to be devised.

In assessing the prospects for final cure it should also be remembered that a proportion of patients will die from complications of therapy, such as intercurrent infections and radiation damage, and that second tumors may subsequently develop. Li et al. observed new malignant tumors in 19 of 414 survivors of childhood cancer.[38] Most were attributable to radiotherapy. These findings emphasize the importance of long-term surveillance in cancer.

Significant improvement in the survival rate has been noted when treatment is carried out in major centers experienced in the management of Wilms' tumor.[8,22,39]

From the foregoing it is apparent that the assessment of prognosis for patients with Wilms' tumor must account for a number of variable features which should be standardized for recording purposes.

1. The staging system should be uniform, and that used by the National Wilms' Tumor Study is recommended. Subclassifications may also be useful, such as size of the tumor, abdominal spill of tumor contents during surgery (which may have different implications from a tumor that is not completely resectable), and sites and multiplicity of metastases (whether to the lungs alone or also to other organs).
2. The histologic features of the tumor should be graded uniformly in all centers. Congenital mesoblastic nephromas should be categorically excluded from the analyses.
3. The age of the patient together with the staging of the disease should be included in the assessment. At present, a demarcation before and after the age of 2 years seems to be most frequently used.
4. The type of therapy employed should be clearly indicated in all reports.

5. The progress assessment of patients at a minimum period of 2 years should indicate separately the proportion of survivors with and without evidence of disease and deaths or complications not attributed to the tumor.

SUMMARY AND CONCLUSIONS

A number of factors related to the prognosis in Wilms' tumor have been analyzed. Patients with Stages I and II disease, histologic types of lesions with differentiated epithelial elements, and children under 2 years of age generally have a better prognosis. The outcome is more favorably influenced by radiotherapy to the primary tumor, at least in more advanced stages of the disease, and to metastatic sites when combined with prolonged chemotherapy. Local recurreneces are uncommon with adequate treatment, and usually appear with metastases elsewhere. The outlook for metastatic disease is improved by combinations of chemotherapy and radiotherapy, with surgical resection of metastases in selected cases. Bilateral Wilms' tumors may be curable in over half of the patients with judicious surgery, radiotherapy, and chemotherapy. Currently, assessment of survival without evidence of disease at 2 years from diagnosis appears to be a valuable guide to the prospects of cure, but may require future revision. Several series have shown the advantage and improved survival when treatment is concentrated in centers experienced with the multidisciplinary management of Wilms' tumors.

With the current forms of treatment available, it is anticipated that the cure rate should be 80 to 90% for localized Wilms' tumor (Stages I and II) and 60 to 70% for metastatic disease.

REFERENCES

1. Garcia, M., Douglass, C., and Schlosser, J. V.: Classification and prognosis in Wilms' tumor. *Radiology* **80**: 574, 1963.
2. Fleming, I., and Pinkel, D.: Clinical staging of Wilms' tumor. *J. Pediatr.* **74**: 324, 1969.
3. Fleming, I. D., and Johnson, W. W.: Clinical and pathologic staging as a guide in management of Wilms' tumor. *Cancer* **26**: 660, 1970.
4. D'Angio, G. J.: Management of children with Wilms' tumor. *Cancer* **30**: 1528, 1972.
5. Currie, D. P., Daly, J. T., Grimes, J. H., and Anderson, E. E.: Wilms' tumor; a clinical pathological correlation. *J. Urol.* **109**: 495, 1973.
6. Margolis, L. W., Smith, W. B., Wara, W. M., et al.: Wilms' tumor; an interdisciplinary treatment program with and without dactinomycin. *Cancer* **32**: 618, 1973.
7. Perez, C. A., Kaiman, H. A., Keith, J., et al.: Treatment of Wilms' tumor and factors affecting prognosis. *Cancer* **32**: 609, 1973.

8. Cassady, J. R., Tefft, M., Filler, R. M., et al.: Considerations in the radiation therapy of Wilms' tumor. *Cancer* **32**: 598, 1973.

9. Maier, J. G., and Harshaw, W. G.: Treatment programs in Wilms' tumor; a study of 51 cases with special reference to the role of actinomycin D. *Cancer* **20**: 96, 1967.

10. Stowens, D.: *Pediatric Pathology*, 2nd ed., Williams and Wilkins, Baltimore, 1966, pp. 658–664.

11. Kenny, G. M., Webster, J. H., Sinks, L. M., et al.: Results from treatment of Wilms' tumor at Roswell Park, 1927–1968. *J. Surg. Oncol.* **1**: 49, 1969.

12. Bannayan, G. A., Huvos, A. G., and D'Angio, G. J.: Effect of irradiation on the maturation of Wilms' tumor. *Cancer* **27**: 812, 1971.

13. Bolande, R. P., Brough, A. J., and Izant, R. J., Jr.: Congenital mesoblastic nephroma of infancy. *Pediatrics* **40**: 272, 1967.

14. Favara, B. E., Johnson, W., and Ito, J. Renal tumors in the neonatal period. *Cancer* **22**: 845, 1968.

15. Wigger, H. J.: Fetal hamartoma of the kidney. *Am. J. Clin. Pathol.* **51**: 323, 1969.

16. Richmond, H., and Dougall, A. J.: Neonatal renal tumors. *J. Pediatr. Surg.* **5**: 413, 1970.

17. Gross, R. E.: *The Surgery of Infancy and Childhood*, W. B. Saunders Company, Philadelphia, 1953.

18. Scott, L. S.: Wilms' tumor; its treatment and prognosis. *Br. Med. J.* **1**: 200, 1956.

19. Sukarochana, K., and Kiesewetter, W. B.: Wilms' tumor; factors affecting long-term survival. *J. Pediatr.* **69**: 747, 1966.

20. Ledlie, E. M., Mynors, L. S., Draper, G. J. and Gormach, P. D.: Natural history and treatment of Wilms' tumour; an analysis of 335 cases occurring in England and Wales, 1962–1966. *Br. Med. J.* **4**: 195, 1970.

21. Farber, S., Toch, R., Sears, E. M., and Pinkel, D.: Advances in chemotherapy of cancer in man. *Adv. Cancer Res.* **4**: 1, 1956.

22. Farber, S.: Chemotherapy in the treatment of leukemia and Wilms' tumor. *JAMA* **198**: 826, 1966.

23. Howard, R.: Nephroblastoma (Wilms' tumour); improved prognosis with actinomycin D. *Med. J. Aust.* **2**: 141, 1964.

24. Colebatch, J. H., Howard, R., Williams, A. L., et al.: Results of actinomycin D therapy for Wilms' tumor. *Int. J. Cancer* **20**: 491, 1964.

25. Fernbach, D. J., and Martyn, D. T.: Role of dactinomycin in the improved survival of children with Wilms' tumor. *JAMA* **195**: 1005, 1966.

26. Wolff, J. A., Krivit, W., Newton, W. A., Jr., and D'Angio, G. J.: Single versus multiple dose dactinomycin therapy of Wilms' tumor; a controlled co-operative study conducted by the Children's Cancer Study Group A. *N. Engl. J. Med.* **279**: 290, 1968.

27. Wolff, J. A., D'Angio, G. J., Hartmann, J., et al. Long-term evaluation of single versus multiple courses of actinomycin D therapy of Wilms' tumor. Prepared by the Children's Cancer Study Group A. *N. Engl. J. Med.* **290**: 84, 1974.

28. Sutow, W. W., Thurman, W. G., and Windmiller, J.: Vincristine (leurocristine) sulfate in the treatment of children with metastatic Wilms' tumor. Pediatric Division, Southwest Cancer Chemotherapy Group. *Pediatrics* **832**: 880, 1963.

29. Sullivan, M. P., Jussey, D. H., and Ayala, A. G.: Wilms' tumour. In Sutow, W. W., Vietti, T. J., Fernbach, D. J. (Eds.): *Clinical Pediatric Oncology*, C. V. Mosby Company, St. Louis, 1973, pp. 359–383.

30. Vietti, T. J., Sullivan, M. P., Haggard, M. E., et al.: Vincristine sulfate and radiation therapy in metastatic Wilms' tumor. *Cancer* **25**: 12, 1970.

31. Martin, J., and Rickham, P. P.: Wilms' tumour, an improved prognosis; report of 22 consecutive children seen from 1967 to 1971. *Arch. Dis. Child.* **49**: 459, 1974.

32. O'Gorman Hughes, D. W., Bowring, A. C., Kern, I. B., et al.: Wilms' tumour; increasing hopes for survival. *Med. J. Aust.* **2**: 917, 1973.

33. Waggett, J., and Koop, C. E.: Wilms' tumor; preoperative radiotherapy and chemotherapy in the management of massive tumors. *Cancer* **26**: 338, 1970.

34. Sullivan, M. P., Sutow, W. W., Cancir, A., and Taylor, G.: Vincristine sulfate in management of Wilms' tumor; replacement of preoperative irradiation by chemotherapy. *JAMA* **202**: 381, 1967.

35. Wedemeyer, P. P., White, J. G., Nesbit, M. E., et al.: Resection of metastases in Wilms' tumor; a report of three cases cured of pulmonary and hepatic metastases. *Pediatrics* **41**: 446, 1968.

36. Ragab, A. H., Vietti, T. J., Crist, W., et al.: Bilateral Wilms' tumor; a review. *Cancer* **30**: 983, 1972.

37. Collins, V. P.: Wilms' tumor; its behavior and prognosis. *J. Louisiana State Med. Soc.* **107**: 474, 1955.

38. Li, F. P., Jaffe, N., and Cassady, J. R.: Risk of second tumors in survivors of childhodd cancer (abstr.). Proceedings of the American Association for Cancer Research and American Society of Clinical Oncology, Houston, March, 1974

39. Sutow, W. W., Chemotherapy in Wilms' tumor; an appraisal. *Cancer* **32**: 1150, 1973.

40. Lemerle, J., and Donaldson, S.: Wilms' tumor; current concepts in diagnosis, prognosis and treatment. *Paediatrician* **1**: 220, 1972–1973.

Author Index

Subject Index

233